Kathleen Pra
7822 79th Ln
Glendale, NY 11385-7450

S0-BYD-697

THE GUILFORD FAMILY THERAPY SERIES
Michael P. Nichols, Series Editor

Recent Volumes

ESSENTIAL ASSESSMENT SKILLS
FOR COUPLE AND FAMILY THERAPY

Essential Assessment Skills for Couple and Family Therapists

LEE WILLIAMS
TODD M. EDWARDS
JoELLEN PATTERSON
LARRY CHAMOW

Series Editor's Note by
MICHAEL P. NICHOLS

THE GUILFORD PRESS
New York   London

© 2011 The Guilford Press
A Division of Guilford Publications, Inc.
72 Spring Street, New York, NY 10012
www.guilford.com

All rights reserved

No part of this book may be reproduced, translated, stored in
a retrieval system, or transmitted, in any form or by any means,
electronic, mechanical, photocopying, microfilming, recording,
or otherwise, without written permission from the Publisher.

Printed in the United States of America

This book is printed on acid-free paper.

Last digit is print number: 9 8 7 6 5 4 3 2 1

The authors have checked with sources believed to be reliable in their
efforts to provide information that is complete and generally in accord
with the stndards of practice that are accepted at the time of publication.
However, in view of the possibility of human error or changes in behavioral,
mental health, or medical sciences, neither the authors, nor the editor and
publisher, nor any other party who has been involved in the preparation or
publication of this work warrants that the information contained herein is
in every respect accurate or complete, and they are not responsible for any
errors or omissions or the results obtained from the use of such information.
Readers are encouraged to confirm the information contained in this book
with other sources.

Library of Congress Cataloging-in-Publication Data is available
from the Publisher.

ISBN 978-1-60918-079-9

About the Authors

Lee Williams, PhD, is Professor of Marital and Family Therapy at the University of San Diego and does couple therapy with veterans at the VA San Diego Medical Center.

Todd M. Edwards, PhD, is Associate Professor and Director of the Marital and Family Therapy Program at the University of San Diego and Assistant Clinical Professor in the Department of Family and Preventive Medicine at the University of California, San Diego.

JoEllen Patterson, PhD, is Professor of Marital and Family Therapy at the University of San Diego and Associate Clinical Professor in the Department of Family and Preventive Medicine and the Department of Psychiatry at the University of California, San Diego.

Larry Chamow, PhD, is Clinical Professor of Marital and Family Therapy at the University of San Diego and is in full-time private practice at the Pacific Family Institute in Carlsbad, California.

Series Editor's Note

One of the hardest things about being a therapist is confronting the burden of other people's troubles. In every first session, a group of worried strangers walk in and hand you their most urgent problem. Someone is depressed, or anxious, or scared, or having trouble controlling his or her anger. The pressure to do something about these painful feelings can be almost overwhelming. That's why for many therapists an assessment is something to get out of the way in order to get down to the business of helping people. You can probably guess that I'm going to say that this is a mistake. If so, you're half right.

A good assessment should help you understand why people are having the problems they're having—and why they haven't been able to solve them. Why is the daughter depressed? Why is the mother upset? And why haven't their families been able to help them? In order to answer these questions, you have to do a little digging—and you have to know where to dig. That's why a book like this one is such a useful addition to any clinician's bookshelf.

In this volume, Lee Williams and his colleagues offer a comprehensive look at the full range of issues anyone making an assessment might want to consider. Some of these issues may be obvious, but many are not. No matter how many clients you've seen, you'll find valuable suggestions for assessment options that you may sometimes overlook.

When I said you'd be half right if you expected me to say that hasty assessments are a mistake, I meant that while you should be thorough, a good assessment need not be a lengthy and formal routine, and it should fit in organically with your style of therapy. If you're considering a psychodynamic approach, for example, many of the typical clinic's arrangements—secretaries making appointments, generic and intrusive questionnaires, and so on—will compromise your chances of creating a confidential relationship. Similarly, while you need to know if one of your clients is using drugs or contemplating suicide, you don't necessarily need to ask every one of them if they do.

When a psychiatrist asks a mildly depressed college student if she hears voices and she says no, this yields a certain amount of information. The psychiatrist learns that the client probably isn't schizophrenic, and she learns that he has no sense of who she is.

When it comes to treating couples and families, a good assessment must explore the presenting complaint while at the same time challenging the family certainty that the problem is located exclusively in the internal machinery of the identified patient. A therapist broadens the focus from the identified patient to relational patterns in a family through a process of probing but respectful questioning. A systemic assessment also explores what family members may be doing to perpetuate the presenting problem. The trick is to help clients see how their actions may be maintaining their problems, without provoking defensive resistance.

In broadening the focus of exploration it's well to remember that the therapist is also part of the system in treatment. Most people—especially people who come to therapy—tend to create certain kinds of problematic relationships in their lives, and they tend to re-create similar relationships with their therapists. Thus, therapists should be alert to transference, countertransference, and projective identification.

Finally, assessments should point toward desired changes. And don't forget to ask yourself, "Desired by whom?" In working with families, the art of assessment is to discover what stands in the way of the family reaching its goals and join with them in a vision of how to get from where they are to where they want to be. After developing a clear and thorough picture of what's keeping a family stuck, and how they got that way, the therapist should talk with them about who needs to change what—and who is willing or unwilling. Without this step, which turns the process of assessment from an operation performed *on* families into an operation performed *with* them, therapy often becomes a process of pushing people where they see no reason to go. No wonder they resist.

These are just some of the issues explored in *Essential Assessment Skills for Couple and Family Therapists*.

MICHAEL P. NICHOLS, PhD

Preface

L earning family therapy can be a challenging enterprise. We originally wrote *Essential Skills in Family Therapy* (Patterson, Williams, Edwards, Chamow, & Grauf-Grounds, 2009) to help our students learn the skills necessary to become effective practitioners. Although assessment is covered in that volume, it primarily focuses on treatment skills. We recognized that there was a lot more we could say about assessment to help our students develop their clinical competence. Thus, we decided to write *Essential Assessment Skills for Couple and Family Therapists* as a companion volume to our original book.

Although the book is primarily written with beginning therapists in mind, we believe more experienced therapists who are learning to work with couples or families will find the book beneficial. The chapters on couples and family assessment will quickly orient the reader to the essential elements that need to be considered in working with couples and families.

This is a unique assessment book in a number of ways. Many other volumes focus heavily or exclusively on using assessment instruments. Although we consider these to be a valuable part of assessment and include them in the book, we recognize that most family therapists rely primarily on the clinical interview for conducting assessments. Thus, the book emphasizes what therapists should explore through clinical interviewing, as well as specific issues or questions to consider within these areas.

Many assessment books focus on a specific problem or population. *Essential Assessment Skills for Couple and Family Therapists* addresses the wide range of issues and populations that family therapists must be equipped to treat. The book not only discusses how to assess couples generally, but also examines special topics (affairs, sexual problems) and specific populations (same-sex couples, premarital couples) that couple therapists are likely to encounter. Similarly, the chapters on assessment of families include unique considerations encountered when working with diverse family types such as stepfamilies, single-parent families, or gay and lesbian families.

Although the book looks at assessment primarily from a systemic perspective, family therapists must also consider the impact of individual functioning on couples and families. Therefore, we include chapters on assessing individual functioning and psychopathology for both adults and children or adolescents. Throughout the book we emphasize the need to simultaneously consider individual and relationship functioning due to their bidirectional influence on one another.

Finally, the present volume is unique in that it considers assessment throughout all phases of therapy. Although most of the book is devoted to assessment issues early in therapy, it also provides guidance on how to take what you have learned from assessment and turn it into a treatment plan. We also discuss how to assess whether clients are making progress in therapy and if they are ready for termination.

Essential Skills in Family Therapy has become a popular text because students find it a practical and readable guide. We have tried to capture that same tone and readability in this book. We use numerous clinical examples to illustrate the concepts. We also include a number of mnemonics throughout the book that students report are helpful in remembering what to include in assessments. We hope and anticipate that the book will be a reference you will go back to again and again. With that goal in mind, we have compiled a list of the mnemonics, assessment techniques, and instruments into an appendix at the end of the book that you can easily refer to at any time.

Contents

ESSENTIAL ASSESSMENT SKILLS
FOR COUPLE AND FAMILY THERAPISTS

CHAPTER 1

Introduction to Assessment

The key to wisdom is knowing all the right questions.
—JOHN A. SIMONE, SR.

Assessment is fundamentally important to therapy. In fact, it could be argued that it is the foundation upon which treatment rests. If the therapy process does not build upon a solid and accurate assessment, attempts to treat our clients can fall apart. The importance of assessment is evident in the number of purposes it serves.

First, assessment helps you uncover what your clients expect from therapy. Obviously this will include what changes they would like to make. It may also include expectations around how therapy will be conducted. Clients may have preconceived notions of how long therapy will last or who will be included. Some clients will expect you to give them homework or specific suggestions, while others will be content simply using you to vent or as a sounding board. Understanding these expectations allows you to negotiate a viable contract for therapy.

Second, assessment helps you understand how problems manifest and impact your clients' lives. Both Rebecca and Jodi report being depressed. However, each is affected by her depression in different ways. Rebecca is moderately depressed, but is able to function adequately at work. Jodi, in contrast, consistently misses days of work because she cannot get out of bed. Rebecca does not have any thoughts of suicide, whereas Jodi often thinks about what it would be like to end her life.

1

Beyond its diagnostic value, assessment can facilitate our joining with clients if it helps us better understand their pain and suffering.

Third, assessment helps you figure out why the problem exists. Why does the couple in front of you constantly fight? Why is the 4-year-old boy prone to angry outbursts and aggression towards his parents? Why is your middle-aged male client depressed? Through assessment, you develop a conceptual understanding of how the problem developed and is maintained. This understanding can help you determine what changes your clients need to make.

The fourth purpose assessment serves is to help you select the best treatment for your clients. Assessment can help you answer the specificity question— which treatment, under what conditions, will offer the best results for this particular client? A therapist working with a depressed woman named Carla recognized through ongoing assessment that she needed to modify her treatment approach. Although the therapist preferred focusing on a client's affect, she learned in one session that Carla had read an article she had found very helpful. The article focused on challenging one's negative thinking. This discussion, in combination with other clues provided during therapy, led the therapist to shift to a more cognitive approach with Carla.

The fifth purpose of assessment is to evaluate how effective therapy is in bringing about change. Have things improved, stayed the same, or perhaps even deteriorated? Assessment can be used to evaluate the effectiveness of a specific intervention or the overall success of therapy. It also aids you in determining when clients are ready for termination.

CHALLENGES OF DOING
AN EFFECTIVE ASSESSMENT

Learning assessment skills as a beginning family therapist can be a challenge. Beginning therapists often question their assessment skills, wondering if they missed something important or asked the right questions. This book walks you through the various areas you need to assess when working with different populations or presenting problems in order to help you be more confident that you are being thorough in your assessment. In addition, we describe specific tools and questions you can use when exploring these different topic areas.

Beginning therapists can feel overwhelmed with the amount of information they obtain from assessment. It may be difficult to prioritize all of the information you have collected, and therefore difficult to know where to focus your clinical energy during treatment. The final chapter of this book will provide you guidance on how to take what you have learned through assessment and shape it into a treatment plan that can guide your work.

Another challenge facing beginning therapists is using theory to inform one's assessment. Theories can help therapists make sense of what they are observing and suggest ways to intervene. Thus, applying theory to both assessment and treatment can be helpful.

One mistake we sometimes see therapists make is to maintain a strong allegiance to a particular theory and apply it to all of their cases. We believe the risk of relying on a single theory is that the therapist will attend only to things that are congruent with that theory and overlook other potentially important factors. A therapist using structural family therapy, for example, may miss the importance of transgenerational issues in a case.

The philosophy of this book is that the appropriate theory for conceptualizing the case will ideally emerge from the assessment data. The best theory to use can depend on a number of different factors, including the presenting issue, underlying causes, client characteristics, and the fit between the therapist's and clients' theories of change. Evidence-based research may also guide the therapist in which approach to use. Therefore, we advocate being able to look at your clients from different theoretical perspectives and then choose the approach that best fits the case. This is not to imply that only one theory will work with a particular case. In many cases, more than one theory could be successfully applied. However, generally speaking, some theories are more fitting than others when conceptualizing a case.

Given this philosophy, the book does not present assessment from one specific theoretical approach. Rather, it attempts to present assessment from an integrative perspective that is compatible with a variety of theories. Obviously, certain questions will be more pertinent to some theories than others. Questions that focus on meaning, for example, will fit better with narrative or cognitive approaches. In contrast, questions that focus on affect will resonate with approaches like emotionally focused therapy. Using our assessment guidelines will provide you with enough information so you can pick the best theory or approach to guide your treatment.

Beginning family therapists can face other challenges that relate to assessment. They sometimes feel pressure to intervene before they have a thorough understanding of the problem and its underlying causes. Although clients in crisis may need immediate intervention, be careful about taking action before you have a clear understanding of the case.

Beginning therapists may also question their ability to accurately diagnose or conceptualize a case due to their lack of experience. As a result, they may be reluctant to share their perspective with other treatment team members (e.g., psychiatrists, case managers). Of course, other therapists may make the opposite mistake, putting too much confidence in their opinions and not being open to other professionals' views.

A BIOPSYCHOSOCIAL-SYSTEMS MODEL

As family therapists, we work primarily from a systems perspective. Essentially this means that we try to understand problems in the context of our clients' relationships. Suzanne, a 38-year-old single mother who is depressed, brings Zachary, her 7-year-old son, to therapy because of his misbehavior. A therapist working from a systemic perspective will observe that Zachary seems to act out in order to get the attention of his mother, who would otherwise be depressed and withdrawn. Including the mother in the formulation and treatment will be necessary to effectively resolve Zachary's behavioral issues.

As systemic therapists, we recognize that our clients often find themselves caught in relational patterns that create problems for them. Devon, for example, feels that Amber is smothering him. He reacts by pulling away and becoming more distant. Amber, in response to his withdrawal, pursues more vigorously in order to fulfill her need for connection. However, her efforts only fuel Devon's sense that he is being smothered. Identifying and altering these interactional patterns is the key to successful therapy.

Even in cases where we could label the person as having an "individual" problem, considering the relational context is still important. Families, for example, do not cause schizophrenia. However, they can and do influence the course of the illness in many individuals. Individuals with schizophrenia are more likely to have relapses if they have family members who are critical, hostile, and intrusive (sometimes referred to as high expressed emotion). Conversely, supportive family members can be a protective factor for individuals with psychopathology.

One mistake we sometimes see beginning family therapists make is putting too much emphasis on individual factors, particularly if only an individual presents for therapy. You need to be constantly asking yourself how the relational context may be shaping your clients' thoughts, feelings, and behavior. Whenever possible, invite the couple or family into therapy, since it is easier to see the relational dynamics in action when family members are present.

Although this book will focus mainly on couples and families as the primary relational system, it is important to acknowledge that systemic principles can be used to understand a variety of other relationships. Systemic principles could be applied to friendships, work relationships, or our clients' relationships with other professionals (e.g., physicians, lawyers, teachers, caseworkers).

Although the systemic approach provides the overarching framework by which we conduct assessment, we recognize that it is important to integrate assessment from other domains. These include biological, psychological, cultural/contextual, and spiritual factors. The biopsychosocial framework (Engel, 1977) reminds us to consider these various areas when doing assessment. Each of these levels can interact together, shaping our clients' experiences. The importance of each of these areas is briefly summarized below.

Biological Factors

Therapists may overlook the role of biology due to their training, which generally focuses on psychological processes. One woman recently described her struggles with depression in a *New York Times* article (Belfort, 2007). The woman went through 4 years of therapy and was treated with multiple medications and shock therapy. All were unsuccessful in resolving her depression. A full blood workup eventually uncovered that she had hyperparathyroidism. The woman's depression has not returned since her hyperparathyroidism was successfully treated. This woman's experience is a stark reminder not to overlook the possibility of organic or biological problems causing what initially appear to be psychological disorders.

Medications can also contribute to or cause psychological problems and need to be ruled out. The onset of Patricia's depression was linked with a change of medication to treat her low blood pressure. When the medication was stopped, her depression immediately began to disappear. Therapists may also encounter individuals who have experienced negative sexual side effects from taking antidepressants.

Health issues or illness can also exacerbate relationship problems. Larry and Sandra successfully worked on a number of different problems to improve their marriage. Although the couple's relationship had significantly improved through these interventions, the couple reported a dramatic improvement in their marriage after Larry's chronic back pain had been successfully treated through a surgical procedure. The chronic pain had led Larry to feel irritable most of the time, which made the couple more prone to conflict.

Psychological Factors

Since couples and families are composed of and created by individuals, psychological factors affecting individuals are important in assessment. The relationship between individuals and a couple or family system is like the relationship between primary and secondary colors. If you wish to create a shade of purple, you must mix red and blue in the proper proportions. In much the same way, two individuals are like primary colors that in combination create a unique relationship dynamic or outcome (e.g., a shade of purple). If you desire a different shade of purple, you don't adjust the color purple directly, but alter the proportion of the primary colors. The process of changing a couple or family system happens in much the same way. You do not change the system directly, but you do it through getting one or more of the individuals in the system to change. Thus, successfully changing a couple or family system requires that you understand each individual within that system.

Assessment can cover a number of psychological factors, but it should evaluate the general domains of affect, behavior, and cognitions. All three are interrelated. Creating change in one domain may lead to change in the other two areas.

Affect (or lack of it) is often a key symptom of psychological disorders such as depression, mania, or schizophrenia. Thus, it can be a critical diagnostic clue in identifying mental illness. Affect can also provide clues as to how an individual is making meaning out of the events in his or her life. Anastasia tried to downplay the impact of the abuse she experienced growing up, but she could not hide the anger and shame she felt when talking about her family of origin.

Assessing behavior can also provide rich insight, such as information on a client's level of functioning. Whether or not your client is able to do the daily tasks of life may help you evaluate the degree to which his or her life is impaired by depression. Observing behavior may also give you clues as to what a client may be thinking or feeling. Joseph would begin to fiddle with his cane whenever he started to become upset by his wife's comments.

Cognitions are also important to explore because they determine how we make sense of the world around us, which in turn determines how we feel and how we interact with the world. Distorted cognitions, for example, can underlie depression. Our cognitions can also impact how we make sense of other family members' behavior, creating the potential for closeness or conflict. After an evening out, Kim said that she was tired and wanted to go to sleep. Ben was interested in some physical contact after they went to bed, so he reached over and put his arm around Kim. When she became irritated, Ben pulled away and got up to go to his computer. When they discussed the incident in therapy both became agitated and began blaming each other. Kim said she thought that whenever Ben touches her he wants sex. Ben said that he just wanted some contact and he felt like she "never wants to be touched."

Careful evaluation of affect, behavior, and cognitions may uncover psychopathology. A potential mistake therapists can make is to miss that a client is struggling with some form of psychopathology. Therapists who work in settings where diagnosing mental illness is minimized or discouraged are most prone to making this mistake. Pay attention to anything that seems unusual or out of the ordinary, and consider whether it may indicate a mental illness. Chapters 6 and 8 specifically address how to assess for psychopathology in adults and children or adolescents.

It is important you take a balanced view between relationship functioning and psychopathology. You want to avoid overlooking a client's psychopathology by focusing exclusively on relationship dynamics. Conversely, you want to avoid the opposite mistake of focusing just on a client's psychopathology, ignoring the role that couple or family relationships have on the etiology or course of the mental illness.

Cultural and Contextual Factors

Cultural and other contextual factors are another important level to consider in assessment. Through socialization, certain beliefs and values can be instilled in an individual by his or her environment. These beliefs and values can influence how individuals relate to one another. Race or ethnicity, for example, can shape the way our clients decide how to balance the collective needs of the family and those of the individual. In addition to race and ethnicity, gender, religious affiliation, sexual orientation, or socioeconomic status may influence our clients' beliefs. Many of these contextual factors may overlap, creating a rich and unique blend of values and beliefs among our clients.

The community or neighborhood in which clients live can be another important contextual factor, impacting your clients' quality of life, in both positive and negative ways. For example, are gangs or crime a concern in the neighborhood? What is the quality of the schools within the community? What is the availability of public transportation, and how does it impact your clients' ability to access jobs or other services?

A mistake that we commonly see beginning therapists make is to overlook cultural or contextual factors in their assessment. You should be asking yourself if there are any important cultural or contextual factors that may be impacting your clients' beliefs or daily life experiences.

Spiritual Issues

Spiritual issues are another important consideration in assessment. How individuals make meaning of things is often shaped or informed by their religious or spiritual beliefs. Roxanne came to therapy to deal with grief issues surrounding the death of her husband. The therapist soon discovered that Roxanne believed her husband had died because God was punishing her. For many clients, however, spiritual or religious beliefs are a source of comfort and strength that therapists may wish to draw upon (Walsh, 2009).

Spirituality or religiosity can also be an important social context for your clients. A client who is involved in a religious community (e.g., church, temple, mosque) can find it to be an important source of social support. Religious socialization can also shape a client's beliefs about marriage or family. Some religions, for example, encourage men and women to adhere to traditional gender roles. Thus, you need to be mindful of the multiple ways in which spiritual issues can play out in a biopsychosocial-systems framework.

SEVEN GUIDING PRINCIPLES OF ASSESSMENT

This book will explore a variety of approaches and questions that you can use to assess a range of clinical issues. However, to increase the effectiveness of your assessment skills, you will need to move beyond a formulaic approach to assessment. Beyond simply asking a set of questions, effective assessment follows certain principles. Using the seven principles described below (see Table 1.1) will enhance your assessment skills.

Joining Is Critical to Assessment

Effective assessment is highly dependent upon the quality of the therapeutic relationship. Clients will be reluctant to disclose sensitive information if they think you do not care, are judgmental, or will use the information against them. If you have a good relationship with your clients, you are more likely to get honest and cooperative responses. Therefore, it is essential that you work to join with your clients as quickly as possible to facilitate assessment in the early stages of therapy. It is also not uncommon for clients to disclose more sensitive information later in therapy after they have developed confidence in the safety of the relationship. Samuel did not initially mention to his therapist that he had delusions of being God until later in therapy when he felt it was safe to disclose this information to her.

Be Curious

One of the greatest assets a therapist can possess is curiosity. Curiosity is important in assessment for at least three reasons. First, curi-

---

TABLE 1.1. Seven Guiding Principles for Conducting Assessment

- Joining is critical to assessment.
- Be curious.
- Think assessment all the time.
- Assessment is intervention, and intervention is assessment.
- Assess for strengths.
- Assessment includes the therapist.
- Assess using multiple perspectives.

osity can encourage us to explore topics more deeply to understand what the client did not immediately see or reveal. This, in turn, can uncover important information that can be essential to understanding the client. During one session, Debra was asked to describe the one important change she would like to see her husband focus on during the week. She refused, stating that she wanted Lance to come up with the behavior. The therapist was curious as to why she took this stance and asked about it further. Debra stated that she wanted him to take responsibility for his actions. When asked to explain why she felt so strongly about this, Debra began to cry and stated that it did not feel safe to ask anything of him. She added that Lance was just like her father, who always blamed her for everything. Due to her experience with her father, Debra was sensitive to any suggestions from Lance that she was to blame for their problems or that he was avoiding taking responsibility for his actions. This proved to be invaluable in helping to uncover part of the interactional cycle that the couple struggled with in their relationship.

Being curious can also encourage us to be less judgmental, which encourages our clients to be more open with us. If we focus solely on the client's behavior, it is tempting to judge whether that behavior is right or wrong, appropriate or inappropriate. Curiosity encourages us to look at the client's underlying motivations or contextual factors that influenced the behavior. Understanding these factors may allow us to have more compassion for the client, even one whose behavior we find offensive (e.g., child abuse, domestic violence). At an agency staff meeting, a supervisor presented the case of a 16-year-old young man who said he had molested his 13-year-old stepsister. He asked the staff who might be interested in working with the case and the room went silent. A discussion ensued among the staff, where they talked about their preconceived ideas about the young man. Their reluctance to work with him stemmed from judgments of his behavior and fears of feeling uncomfortable when sitting with him. The supervisor asked the group to try to detach from their judgments and feelings, and instead to summon their curiosity about the young man. Had someone molested him? What did he mean by "molested"? How did he make sense out of what had occurred? What kinds of problems have been going on in the family? Being curious helped the staff to set aside their judgments and attempt to understand what might be occurring in this case.

Finally, being curious can help us overcome our inhibition about asking difficult questions. Many topics therapists need to be comfortable asking their clients about may violate social norms. It would generally be rude or impolite for a stranger to ask another person about his or her sexual life. Yet, you need to be comfortable asking these types of questions to effectively work with couples. Curiosity helps us overcome that inhibition.

Think Assessment All the Time

Beginning therapists often conceptualize therapy as occurring in distinct phases: it starts with joining and covering administrative issues (e.g., informed consent, confidentiality), proceeds to the assessment phase, and then, after the assessment phase has been completed, treatment can begin.

Although there is some truth to this timeline, it is important to think assessment all the time. After you have formulated a treatment plan, you need to continue assessing the client to help evaluate treatment effectiveness and modify treatment as necessary. Important information can also come out in the earlier phases of therapy before formal assessment has begun, such as when handling routine administrative issues. When his therapist requested permission to videotape sessions for supervision, one client said that he was uncomfortable being taped, hinting at possible involvement in illegal activities.

You should also recognize that during assessment, important information that could be easily overlooked can come out in unexpected ways. In one clinic, couples are routinely given an assessment packet that includes a variety of printed relationship instruments. When a therapist casually asked how completing the battery of assessment instruments had gone, the wife admitted that she experienced great difficulty with it. The therapist then learned that the wife had very limited reading abilities, which easily could have gone unrecognized. In another example, a therapist during a home visit instructed the family to go to the living room so she could do an assessment exercise called a family sculpture. The mother responded, "We've never been in here together as a family." As it turns out, this was an indicator of the family's high level of disengagement. In both examples, important information could have been overlooked if the therapist had narrowly focused only on the results from the relationship inventories or sculpture.

Assessment Is Intervention, and Intervention Is Assessment

A supervisor once said, "Assessment is intervention, and intervention is assessment." Years of clinical experience have proven this principle to be true. In many cases, assessment can be a powerful catalyst for change, even though our intent is not to bring about change through our questions. Questions that you ask can introduce new information to a client or a family system, which in turn can lead to change. During an initial interview, a therapist successfully mapped out the problem cycle with which Scott and Emily struggled. The therapist was surprised to hear the couple report that things had significantly improved since the last session, particularly since the therapist had not attempted to intervene in breaking the couple's cycle. The couple stated that once they saw their cycle on the whiteboard, they knew they needed to find ways to interrupt the cycle, which they did successfully on their own during the week.

Intervention is also assessment. How clients respond to your interventions provides new information that can be incorporated into your understanding of the client or family system. (Remember, think assessment all the time.) In an attempt to deal with a couple's sexual difficulties, the therapist prescribed a sensate focus exercise in which each partner was instructed to touch, caress, and massage the other in ways that would be pleasurable. The person receiving attention was told to give the partner feedback on what was most pleasurable. When it came to doing the exercise at home, the man, contrary to instructions, told his partner not to say anything during her turn. He later reported that he focused on trying to pleasure her in the manner in which he wanted. To his surprise, he became sexually aroused during the exercise. In debriefing why he had altered the sensate focus, the man described how hard he works at trying to please his partner when they do have sex. His response to the exercise helped the man recognize how his preoccupation with pleasing her had prevented him from enjoying the sexual experience himself, which contributed to his low sexual desire. Even a failure to follow a suggestion can provide helpful information, such as potential negative consequences of change.

Assess for Strengths

Therapy often focuses on identifying problems and their causes, making it easy to overlook strengths. However, it is important to assess for both individual and relationship strengths. A couple, for example, might be asked to identify what they like about each other, revealing personal strengths. In addition, they can be asked to comment on relationship strengths, which might include shared personal interests or goals, or compatibility in personalities.

Assessing for strengths is important for a number of reasons. First, identifying strengths can help instill a sense of hope, which may be in short supply in the beginning of therapy. A couple discouraged in their relationship may reconnect with the positive feelings they once felt for one another by talking about how they first met. Second, identifying client strengths can aid you in developing the therapeutic relationship by communicating that you want to see your client in the best possible light, reducing the likelihood he or she will feel judged. Third, strengths can be leveraged to bring about change. A therapist asked Frances, who came to therapy to deal with her husband's recent death, how she had grieved the loss of her parents, who had passed away several years before. Frances was able to describe certain things that helped her deal effectively with the loss of her parents. This provided Frances and her therapist with ideas on how she might successfully cope with her husband's death.

Assessment Includes the Therapist

Some therapists assume that assessment focuses only on the client. Remember that you are part of the therapeutic system. You need to pay attention to your own behaviors and reactions in therapy and assess them just as you do with clients. Nelson, a recently licensed MFT, found himself looking at the clock during much of his session with Mary. The hour seemed to drag, reminding him of when he had recently stood in a long line waiting to buy some tickets. He felt impatient and irritable. He liked Mary, but was tired of listening to her complain about her boyfriend. He wasn't sure how to help her, and it didn't feel like she wanted to change anything. Nelson was bored and was having difficulty concentrating in the session. This was an indication that he was stuck and had lost his sense of direction in therapy.

We need to pay attention when clients elicit strong reactions from us, which may impede therapy. These include finding it difficult to care about or be respectful toward a client, feeling bored and having difficulty concentrating during sessions, feeling helpless and frustrated with a client, having unusual memory lapses regarding the details of the case, and having a very strong positive or negative emotional reaction toward a client.

When you have a strong reaction to a client it is important to assess the impact and the source of these feelings. In terms of impact, are you able to step back from your feelings and maintain objectivity? Is something amiss in the relationship that you and the client should focus upon? In rare cases, it could be that your reaction is so strong that you cannot productively work with that client.

Assessing the source of feelings and reactions is the first step toward gaining some perspective. Is the reaction caused by differences in values or beliefs? Does the client remind you of someone you dislike? Evan admitted that he was having a negative reaction to a female client because she reminded him of his mother, with whom he had a difficult relationship.

Sometimes beginning therapists are quick to assume that their negative reactions to clients reflect issues about themselves. Although this may be true, in many cases it may be more diagnostic of an issue with the client than an issue involving the therapist. Your response could indicate the client has some type of psychopathology (e.g., personality disorder). Or, your reaction may derive from being caught in a parallel process within the client system. In other words, you may find yourself replicating patterns found within the couple or family. As the next vignette illustrates, paying careful attention to your reactions may help you uncover important clues about family dynamics.

Deanne sought supervision regarding her work with a 46-year-old mother who was struggling with parenting her two teenage children. The mother complained that her children did not do as they were told, and were often disrespectful of her. Deanne believed the mother overfunctioned in terms of taking care of her children and had difficulty setting limits with them. Deanne admitted that she was frustrated because the client often talked over her when she attempted to ask a question or make a comment. She also admitted frustration that her client did not seem to follow the multiple suggestions she was offered to improve her parenting. With further discussion, the therapist began to recognize that she and her client were stuck in a pattern similar to that which the client found herself in with her children. Deanne admitted that she was overfunctioning for her client and had difficultly setting limits with her when the client talked over her. Recognizing the parallel process helped

Deanne confirm her initial hypotheses and gave her insight on how to modify her interactions with her client.

Assess Using Multiple Perspectives

The wise clinician will use multiple perspectives when conducting an assessment. Although this may require extra effort on your part, assessing clients from multiple perspectives will help ensure you do not overlook important information. It will also help you determine whether you can trust the information you are gathering. Getting multiple perspectives as a clinician is similar to a journalist getting multiple sources to confirm and deepen a story.

Multiple perspectives can be obtained in different ways. One way is to solicit input from different individuals. One of the principal advantages of family therapy is that you automatically get access to input from multiple individuals. Anyone who has worked with couples will quickly recognize that partners can have very different perspectives on their relationship, with the truth often being a blend of both partners' views. Thus, the therapist who relies only on one person's perspective will end up with a distorted view of the case. In a similar manner, children or adolescents may paint a different picture from their parents or caregivers. Therefore, it is vital to use a variety of sources. Teachers, for example, can provide an important perspective when you work with youth. In other situations, it may be prudent to get input from other professionals (e.g., caseworkers, therapists) or individuals (e.g., extended family, friends) who can offer additional insight about the individual, couple, or family.

It is also wise to use various methods of assessment as a means of obtaining multiple perspectives. Various forms of assessment offer different types of data, each with its own strengths and limitations. Assessment instruments offer quantitative data, whereas the clinical interview offers data that is more qualitative in nature. Generally, using multiple methods will provide data that complement each other, providing a better understanding of our clients. In the first interview, Brady and Susan failed to disclose their concerns regarding their sexual relationship. However, both acknowledged concerns about their sexual relationship on an inventory that assessed marital quality. When asked further about this in the subsequent session, the couple admitted that it was indeed a significant area of concern. In the next chapter we discuss various approaches to collecting assessment information, including the potential strengths and limitations of each.

CONCLUSION

This chapter has described the goals and challenges of doing an effective assessment. It has also articulated the importance of using a biopsycho-social-systems perspective in assessment. The remainder of the book shows in greater detail how this framework can be applied when assessing individuals, couples, and families. Finally, we have described seven guiding principles that we recommend therapists follow to enhance their effectiveness in conducting assessments.

CHAPTER 2

Tools for Assessment

This book will provide you with a blueprint for conducting assessment with a variety of populations and issues. However, getting the information you need requires not only a blueprint to follow, but also tools for assessment. This chapter focuses on four of them: clinical interviewing, assessment instruments, behavioral observation, and physiological assessment. Two of these tools, clinical interviewing and assessment instruments, deserve special attention. They are like a hammer and screwdriver: essential tools in one's assessment toolbox. Therefore, this chapter offers detailed guidelines for using them.

METHODS OF ASSESSMENT

Clinical Interviewing

Asking questions through the clinical interview is the primary tool therapists use for assessment. Many clinical questions ask clients to report on their own thoughts, feelings, or behaviors, but they may also ask clients to comment on what they observe others doing or speculate about what others are thinking or feeling. Although a client's behavior may give us clues to what he or she is thinking or feeling, asking our clients directly can give us the most accurate picture. We also rely on clients to report behaviors that occur in private and cannot be directly observed.

However, the value of clinical questions depends upon the client being cooperative, insightful, and honest, three conditions that may not always be met. Clients will not always be cooperative in answering questions. The sullen teenager dragged to therapy by his parents may refuse to answer questions posed in the first session. Clients may also vary in their levels of insight. Some will have little or no awareness, while others will be introspective and insightful.

You cannot always count on your clients to be honest. Individuals who have sexually abused a child, for example, may deny doing so out of fear of going to jail. A client may also withhold information for fear of getting caught in a lie. Upon being discovered by his wife for having an affair, one man denied having had sex with another woman and insisted that they just had an emotional bond. In spite of evidence to the contrary, he continued to deny the truth in order to avoid further damage. He also withheld the information from the therapist. When the man finally acknowledged that he had slept with the woman, his wife disclosed that she knew he had had another affair earlier in their marriage. Obviously, withholding this kind of critical information in therapy severely impedes progress.

Social desirability, a human being's wish to be looked at in a favorable light, may also keep individuals from being completely truthful. It leads them to overreport positive behaviors or underreport negative behaviors such as substance abuse or violence (Bradburn, Sudman, & Wansink, 2004). Therefore, social desirability may impact a therapist's ability to get a completely accurate picture. It is not unusual for clients with a drinking or drug problem to minimize their substance use even to themselves. A client may truly believe that he only has two or three drinks a night, though in fact he has four or five.

Therapists attempt to deal with social desirability (or honesty in general) in a variety of ways. Offering confidentiality and establishing a safe and nonjudgmental relationship are key. At times, it may be helpful to remind clients that you can be most effective in helping them if they are honest or open about what is happening in their lives. How questions are asked, which is addressed in a later section, can also encourage clients to answer questions more honestly.

Assessment Instruments

Assessment instruments or pencil-and-paper tests can supplement the information gained through clinical interviews. Assessment instruments possess many of the same benefits and limitations as clinical interviews because they both rely on self-report. Thus, assessment instruments are good at providing information on the thoughts, feelings, and behaviors to which only the client has direct access. However, you must also rely on the client to be cooperative, honest, and insightful when completing the instruments.

Despite their similarities, assessment instruments offer unique advantages over clinical questioning. First, they can provide a quick and efficient means of collecting a lot of information. It takes considerably less time for a client to read and mark answers on a questionnaire than to respond verbally to a therapist asking questions. Client responses to interviewer questions are seldom as concise as those offered on an assessment instrument.

Second, assessment instruments provide quantitative data that can be helpful in clinical decision making. Two individuals may both express that they feel depressed. However, their scores on a depression inventory may reveal that one is mildly depressed, whereas the other is severely depressed. A referral for possible medication is definitely warranted for the severely depressed client, whereas the mildly depressed client may not require a referral.

Third, standardization of the questions is another advantage of assessment instruments. Questions are asked in the same way each time, allowing one to compare answers across time or across individuals. Comparing answers over time allows us to see if change or improvement is occurring. Comparing answers across individuals allows us to see how a client's functioning compares to that of others. For example, does the client's score for marital satisfaction fall in the range for those who are seeking therapy for distressed marriages, or is it closer to scores for nonclinical couples?

Fourth, assessment instruments can help us be more thorough in our assessment. Assessment instruments are often evaluated for content validity, which determines if all the salient aspects of the concept being measured are included. Before using an instrument for assessing a disorder, for example, we would want to know if it included all the important symptoms of the disorder. Using the Beck Depression Inventory, which has good content validity, would give us confidence that we have not overlooked an important symptom of depression in our assessment.

Finally, some clients have an easier time disclosing sensitive information through an assessment instrument than they do talking directly about it with a therapist. A couple may first report sexual problems or acts of physical aggression via an assessment instrument rather than volunteer this information in a session.

Assessment instruments also have potential disadvantages. First, answering questions on an inventory is an impersonal experience. Clients may not find it as engaging or as enjoyable as talking with the therapist. Second, clients may feel that not all the questions apply to them. They may be confused or irritated by questions that do not seem to apply. In contrast, it is easier in a clinical interview to modify or tailor questions to a client's situation. Third, assessment instruments typically offer a narrow range of answers (e.g., never, sometimes, often, always), which the client may feel is constricting. Open-ended questions, in contrast, allow the client to answer in any manner that he or she chooses. They also allow the client to provide more detail, offering a richer perspective than an assessment instrument can provide. On an assessment instrument the client would simply report how often she had thoughts of suicide. However, she could not offer her perspective on what was different about the times when she had these thoughts versus times when she did not.

Usually the best approach is to use a combination of clinical interviewing and assessment instruments. A judicious use of assessment instruments, particularly for areas that are routinely evaluated (e.g., marital quality for couples, symptoms of depression), can make assessment more efficient. The data obtained from assessment instruments can be a springboard for exploring topics in more depth through clinical interviewing.

Observation of Behavior

You can gain valuable clinical information about your clients simply by observing them. Behavioral observation can range from informal observations to formal measurement of behavior using coding systems. On the informal end of the spectrum, your observation of client behavior is spontaneous rather than planned or deliberate. You might notice, for example, that a 13-year-old daughter responds to her younger brother's need to go to the bathroom during the session even though his request was initially directed to his mother (and subsequently ignored). Thus, you might suspect that the daughter is parentified.

On the other end of the spectrum, you may deliberately measure a client's behavior using an observational tool. The Beavers Interactional Scales are an example of an observational measure that can be used clinically with families (Hampson & Beavers, 2007). Families are instructed to discuss for 10 minutes what they would like to see changed in their family. The clinician then evaluates the family interactions using various criteria or rating scales. The results can be used to classify families into one of seven family types based on the Beavers model.

Behavioral observation may fall in between these two extremes. You may deliberately create a situation to observe how clients behave (e.g., an enactment), but stop short of using a coding system to formally measure their actions. For example, parents might be instructed to deal with a child who is acting out in session. You then carefully observe what each parent does. Does one parent take the role of disciplinarian while the other silently watches? Does the child obey, resist, or ignore the parent's attempt to correct his or her behavior?

The key advantage of behavioral observation is that it may more accurately reflect what an individual is thinking or feeling compared to what is being spoken. This is because nonverbal communication is under less conscious control than verbal communication. Therefore, if a client's nonverbal and verbal messages are not congruent, pay careful attention to what the nonverbal message is.

However, the key disadvantage of behavioral observations is that we may not always accurately infer the motivations, thoughts, or feelings behind the behavior. It may be obvious, for example, that a loved one is upset based on his or her behavior (e.g., slamming doors), but it may not be clear as to why he or she is upset, or with whom. When discussing a recent conflict in which her partner had been verbally abusive, Charlene became upset. It would be natural to assume that Charlene was upset with her partner's behavior. However, when the therapist checked in with Charlene, she reported being upset at herself for allowing him to treat her in this manner. Therefore, check your inferences with your client to confirm you are getting an accurate picture.

Behavioral observations are often key to uncovering the interactional patterns of a family or couple. Often couples or families reenact their interactional patterns in session, allowing us to observe them first hand. Identifying and interrupting these negative interactions is often the focus of our work with couples and families.

Physiological Measures

Measuring physiological processes is another approach that can be used in assessment. Often this type of assessment will be performed by a medical professional who is attempting to rule out a medical condition. For example, a physician may order blood work be done to rule out hypothyroidism or other possible causes for a client's depression. Urine testing to screen for substance abuse is another way physiological measures might be helpful in therapy. In some cases, a therapist might measure a physiological process during a therapy session, such as using biofeedback. Gottman (1999, pp. 232–233) describes using various methods of measuring heart rates in sessions with couples to help individuals assess if they have diffuse physiological arousal (DPA), which can have an impact on how couples interact.

GUIDELINES FOR ASKING QUESTIONS

Given the heavy reliance that clinicians place on asking questions during assessment, it is important to know how to ask good questions. The following guidelines will help you in constructing effective questions.

Open and Closed Questions

It is important to consider whether your question should be open or closed. Open questions encourage the client to offer a description rather than a brief one- or two-word answer. Closed questions provide the client with choices or imply a choice such as yes or no. An open question might be phrased as "How have the problems in your relationship impacted your commitment to the marriage?" In contrast, a closed version of the question might ask, "Have the problems in the relationship led you to consider divorce?"

Each type of question has potential strengths and limitations. Open questions are generally best when exploring a new topic or getting to know a person. They give the client answering the question the freedom to respond in a manner that makes the most sense to him or her. In other words, they allow the client to guide where the conversation should go, which is appropriate in the beginning as you attempt to learn about your client's concerns, goals, and experiences. In contrast, closed questions require that you know enough about the client's experience to offer appropriate choices, knowledge that you may not possess early in the therapy process. Thus, you should be using a lot of open questions during initial assessment.

Closed questions provide the client clear direction on what the therapist is looking for because the choice of answers is given or clearly implied. Closed questions are usually easier to answer. There are two potential concerns with closed questions, however, that should be kept in mind. First, they can discourage clients from providing much of a description or explanation, which may prevent important information from being disclosed. Second, they presume that the therapist knows enough to offer appropriate responses, which may not always be the case. Prematurely asking a closed question without offering all the appropriate choices may expose the therapist's lack of knowledge about the client or potential biases. A therapist who asks if a client is married may be presuming the individual is heterosexual, which may not be the case.

When asking open or closed questions, you also need to monitor the client's anxiety level in session. Some anxiety is appropriate and is often helpful in motivating change. However, if anxiety gets too high, the client may wish to leave the session or terminate therapy. In general, closed questions will lower a client's anxiety, while open-ended questions will increase it. A question designed to gather specific data or information (such as "How many family members do you have?") is a closed question which the client knows the answer to, so it will lower anxiety. An open question (such as "If you continue to feel this depressed, how do you imagine it will impact your child?") will likely increase the client's anxiety.

Sometimes therapists will fall into the trap of asking a lot of closed questions with clients who are uncooperative or nonexpressive. Since closed questions require less effort to answer, clinicians often have more success in getting these clients to respond to these questions. However, the danger of falling into this pattern is that it permits the client to provide minimal disclosure and forces the therapist to guess (sometimes accurately, sometimes not) what may be going on in the client's life.

Asking Clear Questions

Obviously one wants to ask questions the client understands. You should keep in mind possible factors that may make it difficult for your client to comprehend your question. First, you should ask only one question at a time. Sometimes we will ask about two things at the same time. The question "How happy are you in your marriage, and have you thought about divorce?" asks about two different things (marital satisfaction and divorce).

Second, we need to use language that our clients understand. You should avoid clinical terms or jargon with which the client may be unfamiliar. Clients may not understand if you ask them about boundaries, a term that is familiar to most therapists. Your vocabulary level should also match that of your clients. Unfortunately, clients may not always admit that they do not understand an unfamiliar word. If possible, it is ideal to use your client's language when asking questions.

Third, we need to avoid asking questions that may be difficult for individuals due to their age or intellectual functioning. Young children may have difficulty with questions that are more abstract because they are more concrete in their thinking. In some cases, this may also be true of adults. Suzanne, for example, had difficulty answering questions unless they were very concrete. Her difficulty with questions that required any level of abstract thinking was likely due to the stroke that she had had a year ago, which diminished her intellectual functioning.

Minimizing Social Desirability

As discussed earlier, social desirability may influence how individuals answer questions, underreporting negative behaviors and overreporting positive behaviors. A number of different strategies can be used to encourage clients to more accurately report their behaviors.

One way to reduce underreporting of behaviors that are linked to social desirability (Bradburn et al., 2004) is to "assume" them. One agency found that when screening men for sexual behavior that put them at greater risk for contracting HIV, men were more likely to admit to sexual acts with other men when the behavior was presumed ("How many men have you performed sexual acts with?"), than when they were asked whether they had ever had sexual acts with other men. Although some clients may be bothered by this assumption, they can always answer that they do not engage in that type of behavior.

Another approach is to provide a rationale or normalize the behavior before asking how often an individual engages in it (Bradburn et al., 2004). For example, a therapist might preface a question about alcohol use by saying, "Many people use alcohol socially or to deal with stress or unwind." Statements like these give clients greater permission to admit to these behaviors since others do it.

There is also some evidence from survey research that suggests using an individual's own words or language reduces underreporting of socially undesirable behavior (Bradburn et al., 2004). So, if your client uses the phrase "getting wasted," then it would be best to use this language when inquiring as to how often the individual becomes intoxicated.

When asking about the frequency of a socially undesirable behavior through a closed question, it is important to offer a sufficient range of responses. For example, you might ask if an individual has one, five, 10, or 15 drinks a day. An individual who consumes five drinks a day will be more likely to endorse this amount since it does not appear extreme given these choices. In contrast, if you ask if the individual consumes one, two, or five drinks a day, the individual will be less likely to admit to having five drinks a day, since this is the extreme given the offered choices.

GUIDELINES FOR USING ASSESSMENT INSTRUMENTS

Selecting Instruments

As stated earlier, there is merit in including a judicious number of instruments in clinical assessment. Assessment instruments can be obtained from a variety of sources. Table 2.1 lists books that offer a compilation of assessment instruments for measuring couples and families. Assessment instruments can sometimes be located by searching journal articles or purchased from the companies that publish them. Although some of the measures will have been originally constructed for research purposes, many can be applied to clinical use.

How do you decide what instruments to include? The primary factor to consider is how clinically useful the information will be. Instruments that measure level of functioning for individuals or relationships are frequently helpful. Instruments that help you identify symptoms and reach a possible diagnosis can also be invaluable to clinicians. What the instrument measures should be consistent with how you conceptualize therapy. Possible instruments you may want to use will be suggested throughout the book and are also summarized in the Appendix.

TABLE 2.1. Sourcebooks for Family Therapy Assessment Instruments

- *Assessment of Couples and Families: Contemporary and Cutting-Edge Strategies* (Sperry, 2004)
- *Family Assessment: A Guide to Methods and Measures* (Grotevant & Carlson, 1989)
- *Family Assessment: Resiliency, Coping, and Adaptation: Inventories for Research and Practice* (McCubbin, Thompson, & McCubbin, 1996)
- *Handbook of Family Measurement Techniques* (Vols. 1–3) (Touliatos, Perlmutter, & Straus, 2001)
- *Handbook of Measurements for Marriage and Family Therapy* (Fredman & Sherman, 1987)
- *Measures for Clinical Practice: A Sourcebook. Vol. 1. Couples, Families, and Children* (4th ed.) (Fischer & Corcoran, 2007)
- *Sourcebook of Marriage and Family Evaluation* (L'Abate & Bagarozzi, 1993)
- *The Couple and Family Clinical Documentation Sourcebook: A Comprehensive Collection of Mental Health Practice Forms, Inventories, Handouts, and Records* (Patterson, 1999)

An instrument's clinical value also depends on your ability to interpret what the scores mean. Ideally cutoffs or norms are available for an instrument so you can determine if the score falls in the normal or clinical range or in which percentile the score falls. Scores from an instrument that does not have cutoffs or norms will more be more difficult to interpret, but may still be useful, especially if it is given over time to demonstrate whether the client has changed.

When selecting an assessment instrument to use, you need to evaluate if the instrument is psychometrically sound. An instrument must be both reliable and valid to be psychometrically sound. The simplest way to think of reliability is as a measure of consistency. Different forms of reliability look at different aspects of consistency.

Pencil-and-paper instruments must have good internal reliability. Internal reliability measures if the items within a scale are consistent in measuring a single concept or construct. An instrument intended to measure depression, for example, should not include items that measure other constructs, such as anxiety. All of the items should strongly correlate with one another if a scale has strong internal reliability. Internal reliability is typically reported as a Cronbach's alpha, although a split-half method is sometimes used. The Küder–Richardson, a variation of the Cronbach's alpha, is used for scales composed of dichotomous items (e.g., yes/no). In each of these cases, values of .80 and above are generally considered acceptable, although higher reliabilities (.90 and above) are desirable since these instruments are being used to make decisions about people's lives.

Test–retest reliabilities are sometimes reported for a pencil-and-paper instrument, which evaluates if the scale gives consistent results over time. This is determined by giving the instrument at two different points in time to the same set of people and then seeing if the scores strongly correlate. If a test–retest reliability is reported, it will ideally be .80 or above.

If you use an observational measure or coding system, then the appropriate reliability to consider is interrater reliability. A reliable coding system should produce consistent results across raters. Thus, there should be a strong agreement or correlation between two raters coding the same thing. Interrater reliabilities should generally be .75 and above, although some subscales may have lower values.

In addition to being reliable, an instrument must also be valid. Validity assesses whether an instrument measures what it is supposed to. An instrument can be reliable but consistently give the wrong answer. A variety of methods are used to establish validity. The more methods used, the more confidence one can have in the instrument's validity.

Content validity is a form of validity based on judgment. It is typically established by having experts examine the instrument to ensure the items apply and that important aspects of the construct are not being overlooked.

Criterion validity is demonstrated by showing that the instrument's scores correlate with or predict some chosen (criterion) variable. There are different forms of criterion validity, including predictive, discriminant, and concurrent. Predictive validity evaluates an instrument's ability to accurately predict something in the future (e.g., GRE scores predict graduate school performance). Discriminant validity measures whether an instrument can discriminate between two groups expected to be different (e.g., scores on a marital quality inventory should be different for distressed and nondistressed couples). It is sometimes referred to as known-groups validity. Concurrent validity assesses whether the instrument correlates with another measure of the same construct that has already been established as a valid measure.

Construct validity attempts to demonstrate that the instrument's scores relate with other measures in the way that one would theoretically expect. Construct validity is supported when an instrument correlates with other constructs as anticipated (sometimes called convergent validity). Conversely, the instrument's scores should not correlate with other constructs where a correlation is not expected (sometimes called divergent validity).

Length is another consideration in selecting which instruments to use. Longer instruments will take more time to complete and possibly to score. You will need to weigh this against the potential value of the additional information longer instruments often provide. For example, will a 150-item measure of marital quality (Marital Satisfaction Inventory–Revised) give substantially better information than one with 32 items (Dyadic Adjustment Scale [DAS]) or three items (Kansas Marital Satisfaction Scale)? The answer may depend upon on how the clinician uses the information. A clinician who is simply interested in an overall sense of marital satisfaction will likely be content with a briefer measure. A clinician who is interested in a more detailed picture will be able to glean more information from a longer scale by looking at subscale scores or responses to individual items. In some cases, you could elect to administer one or more subscales rather than the entire instrument.

Other practical considerations may determine whether to use an instrument. Cost may be an important factor. Some instruments can be copied or used with the developer's permission at no cost. Others may need to be purchased in compliance with copyright laws. Obviously free or inexpensive instruments are desirable, especially for students or agencies that have limited financial resources. However, using instruments that need to be purchased may still be justified in certain cases, especially if they are relatively inexpensive. Instruments available for purchase may offer advantages such as being professionally designed, and having manuals to assist in scoring or interpretation, or other scoring aids (e.g., templates, computer programs).

You will also need to determine if you have the proper training to administer and interpret an instrument. In some cases, you may need to show that you have the proper training before you can purchase an instrument. This may require documenting you have taken the necessary coursework or workshops that prepare individuals for administering and interpreting these instruments.

Ease of scoring can be another important factor. Therapists may be discouraged from using instruments that are difficult or time consuming to score or that must be sent to someone else to score for a fee. For instruments that are self-scored, it may be possible to facilitate scoring by creating a spreadsheet that automatically calculates (and perhaps even graphs) the results. An initial investment in time to create the spreadsheet may save significant time in scoring the instruments in the future.

In addition to these general considerations, you will need to determine on a case-by-case basis if an instrument is appropriate for a particular client. An instrument used in a battery of tests may not apply to all clients. For example, the Marital Status Inventory, which measures steps toward divorce, may not apply to a cohabitating couple. There are other factors to consider: Does the instrument fit the reading or comprehension level of the client? Is the client similar enough to the population upon which instrument norms or cutoffs were determined? If not, the results may not give an accurate picture for this particular client.

Administering Assessment Instruments

You should become familiar with an instrument before administering it. An excellent way to do this is for you to administer the instrument to yourself. This will give you insight into what the experience may be like for your client. Questions you find difficult to understand or answer may present a similar challenge to your client. If you can anticipate these problems, you can advise your client on how to best deal with them. Naturally, the more you use an instrument, the better understanding you will have of its strengths and limitations.

When you administer an inventory or battery of instruments to a client, it may be helpful to keep the mnemonic RICE in mind. The first step is to give your clients a *rationale* as to why they are being asked to complete the instruments. The rationale does not need to be extensive or lengthy, but should concisely state why the instruments will be helpful to the therapy process. A couple might be told, for example, that the battery of instruments will help the therapist evaluate the couple's relationship in a number of important areas of couple functioning. The therapist might add that completing the inventories will make the assessment more efficient than asking the couple each of these questions through a clinical interview.

Second, clients should be given clear *instructions* on what is expected of them. A couple might be told, for example, to complete the inventories without consulting their partner. Clients should also

Rationale, Instructions, Confidential, Evaluate

be clearly told when and to whom the instruments should be returned, particularly if they are asked to complete them at home. You should also confirm that the instructions printed on the assessment instruments are clear and easily understood.

Clients will sometimes have questions about who will see the results. Therefore, you may need to reassure clients that the information collected from assessment instruments will be treated in a *confidential* manner similar to other information discussed in therapy. If an instrument must be sent away for scoring, you can discuss the steps taken to assure the client's identity is kept confidential.

Finally, you should *evaluate* your client's response to your request. Generally clients will agree to a request to complete assessment instruments. Thus, pay careful attention to clients who seem reticent or refuse to complete them. Uncovering the reason why can be diagnostic. One woman who expressed concerns about completing the inventory disclosed that she had difficulty with reading due to a recent stroke. Language fluency may be another barrier to completing inventories. Resistance to filling out instruments may also indicate other issues, such as ambivalence about therapy or distrust of others (especially around issues of confidentiality).

Interpreting Results from Assessment Instruments

There are a number of guidelines that you should follow when interpreting results from assessment instruments. Following these guidelines will help ensure the conclusions drawn from the instruments are valid and clinically useful.

Prior to scoring the instrument, you should confirm your client answered all of the questions. Missing responses can affect the scores and interpretation of results. Individuals who fail to answer questions on a marital quality inventory, for example, may appear more distressed because scores for these questions were not added to the total score. It may also be helpful to determine why a question was not answered. Was the question simply overlooked? Or was it left blank because the client did not understand the question or felt it did not apply?

It is a good idea to ask your clients if they had any questions or concerns after filling out the instrument(s). Sometimes the feedback is illuminating and can uncover important clinical information. One couple stated they had difficulty knowing how to answer the questions because the relationship had its ups and downs. This led the therapist to explore from a solution-focused perspective what was different about the times when the relationship was doing well.

When interpreting results, it is often helpful to examine specific items in addition to the total score. For example, the question on suicide ideation on a depression inventory can be important to look at. Examining individual items on a marital quality instrument can help you identify specific problems in the couple's relationship, such as sex, finances, or issues of commitment. Ted's response to a question on commitment on the Dyadic Adjustment Scale reflected his strong ambivalence about being in the marriage, something he had not volunteered in the initial session in order to protect his partner's feelings.

If cutoffs or norms are available, you should determine if the sample upon which the instrument's norms or cutoffs were established is representative of your client. Norms for an instrument based on a white, middle-class sample, for example, should be applied to culturally diverse individuals with caution.

When you present the results of the assessment instrument(s) to your client, it is wise to ask if he or she agrees with the results. If the client disagrees, he or she may be able to provide additional information that puts the results in a different light. One engaged couple who took a premarital inventory was surprised to see their scores were so low. It was discovered that the man had misunderstood how to answer the questions due to his difficulty with English.

Results from assessment instruments should also be considered in relationship to other information about the client. Are the results consistent with other observations of the client? How do the results fit into the overall impression of the client gained from clinical interviewing? If there are contradictions, you should explore what these inconsistencies mean.

Family members should be asked not to use the results of the inventories in a negative or critical way. Therapy needs to be a safe place, and information that is provided should not be used by clients as ammunition to hurt each other.

CONCLUSION

This chapter has described four important methods of assessment: clinical interviewing, assessment instruments, behavioral observation, and physiological measurement. Since clinicians rely so heavily on the clinical interview in assessment, we have described guidelines for how to construct or ask questions. In addition, we have described important considerations for selecting, administering, and interpreting assessment instruments. The skillful use of these methods will enhance your assessment skills. Subsequent chapters examine how these methods can be applied to the assessment of adults, children and adolescents, families, and couples. First, however, we discuss assessment during the initial interview (Chapter 3) and how to assess for safety issues (Chapter 4).

The Initial Interview

Nicole carefully rereads the intake form that her supervisor has just given her. This will be Nicole's first case, a family. Eric and Elizabeth are bringing their 5-year-old son, Nathan, in for therapy. The parents complain their son is having temper tantrums at home. The school also reports he is showing aggressive behavior with his classmates and has difficulty staying in his seat in class. Nicole is quite nervous as she anticipates her first case. Several questions swirl around in her mind. Will they notice she is so inexperienced? Will they question her ability to help them because she is single and does not have children herself? Where should she begin in terms of asking the family questions about their goals for therapy? Will she ask the right questions to begin to formulate a conceptualization of the case?

Nicole's anxiety and the questions she has as she approaches her first session are normal and to be expected for beginning therapists (Patterson, Williams, Edwards, Chamow, & Grauf-Grounds, 2009). Having a clear map of the key tasks she needs to accomplish will help Nicole get through her first session. One of these key tasks is to successfully join with the family. The family will be much more likely to return for a second session if they feel a strong connection with Nicole. Joining is also important for assessment. Clients are more likely to be honest and disclose more information if they feel their therapist understands them and is not judging them. Fortunately, most beginning therapists have confidence in their ability to join with clients because they possess strong relationship skills prior to entering the field. They feel comfortable about being able to listen empathically to individuals as they share their struggles or problems.

The initial session is also the time to handle administrative issues. Going over administrative issues in the beginning of the session provides structure and sets expectations regarding the therapy process. Addressing issues of confidentiality is an essential part of this process. Like joining, confidentiality has implications for assessment. Confidentiality makes it easier for clients to share sensitive information because they have assurance that it will remain private. However, clients need to be made aware that there are certain limits to confidentiality, especially as it relates to others being harmed (e.g., child abuse, suicide, threats of harm to others). The initial session is also the usual time to establish fees for therapy and discuss the therapy process, videotaping, and expectations for attendance. These topics should also be included on a written informed-consent form.

After going over administrative issues, the therapist can begin the initial assessment, which is the focus of this chapter. Initial assessment includes a variety of areas that are generally explored with all clients regardless of whether they present as an individual, couple, or family. Obviously assessing your clients' presenting problems and goals for therapy are important. Initial assessment also includes exploring your clients' motivation for therapy, previous attempts to solve the problems, potential concerns about therapy or the therapist, and client strengths and resources. Subsequent chapters focus on more specific issues such as assessing for safety (e.g., abuse, suicidality) or issues unique to working with individuals, couples, or families.

Before continuing, however, it is important to restate the importance of thinking assessment all the time. Valuable information may come out during each phase of the initial interview. In fact, assessment may begin even before your clients are in the therapy room. In one case, a therapist discovered a husband and wife sitting in opposite parts of the waiting room, which foreshadowed the couple's level of disengagement.

Important information can come out during the introductory phase when you and your clients are getting acquainted. Initial impressions of clients, although tentative, can often be diagnostic. How do the individuals present? Do they seem guarded, nervous, hostile, or depressed? Where do family members sit relative to each other? This may indicate potential alliances or coalitions within the family.

Likewise, addressing administrative issues can uncover important information. A client who asks you a number of questions about your background or age may be subtly (or not so subtly) questioning your credibility. Establishing fees can quickly uncover financial stressors that clients may be experiencing. Questions or concerns about confidentiality may point to hidden agendas or reveal other issues. A husband or wife who asks if the courts can access therapy records may already be thinking of divorce and anticipating a potential child custody battle. Obviously further questioning and observation are needed to determine if initial impressions or hypotheses are valid, but they provide an excellent starting point for assessment.

The general rule of thumb is to pay attention to any reaction or question that seems out of the ordinary. If a client adamantly refuses to be videotaped, then this should be explored further since most clients agree to this if it is presented in a proper fashion. Some clients are simply self-conscious, such as the young woman who was initially reluctant to be taped because she feared individuals watching the tape would judge her. One man who would not allow taping described his fear that the government would get his tapes and spy on him, clearly evidence of delusional thinking. Another man who refused to be taped implied that he had been engaged in illegal activity.

WHAT IS THE PROBLEM?

We typically begin assessment by asking clients what problems are bringing them to therapy. It is important that you hear from everyone in the room when working with a couple or family since each person may have a different perspective. Parents may feel their adolescent son or daughter is irresponsible, while the adolescent feels the parents are too restrictive. Family members may even disagree on whether a problem exists. One mother brought her son to therapy over concerns regarding his behavior. When the father was asked about his son in a subsequent session, he flatly stated that his son's behavior was normal and that no problem existed.

When exploring presenting problems, it is wise to investigate who, what, when, where, and why. Who is seen as having the problem? In many families, one person may be identified as having the problem, often a child. Couples often blame each other for the problems in the relationship. In other cases, however, the problem may be defined more relationally, such as a couple having communication problems, or a family stating they have difficulty getting along with one another.

Another important who question is "Who else knows about the problem?" The answer may help you identify important people in the client's social network. It may also illuminate possible feelings of shame if the client has not told anyone else about the problem. Asking who knows of the problem may also uncover other professionals (e.g., teachers, physicians, therapists) with whom you may need to collaborate. In some cases, the client may disclose that child protective services or the legal system is involved.

Clients sometimes describe problems in rather vague terms, such as "we fight" or "we are having problems communicating." Probing further by asking for a behavioral description of the problem can give you a clearer picture. For example, you might ask if the couple ever yells or puts each other down. Do they ever get physical with one another?

In some cases, it may be important to know where the problem occurs. When working with children, does the problem occur at home, at school, or in both settings? Knowing a problem exists in only one setting may help you narrow down possible causes. Bree, an 11-year-old girl, presented with symptoms of moodiness, withdrawal, and lethargy. Further exploration revealed these symptoms were apparent only when she was at home. Her teacher described Bree as "positive, involved in classroom activities, and interested in her classmates." It seemed that her symptoms occurred only at home in response to her parents' arguing and marital conflict.

Knowing when the problem first arose is also vital information. Is the problem long-standing, or has it recently emerged? Identifying when the problem began may help you uncover a precipitating event, which may give you insight into why the problem came to be. Anthony, a 16-year-old teen, began to use drugs when he was 13. The onset of his drug use coincided with the separation (and eventual divorce) of his parents. If the problem has been long-standing, then it is important to inquire as to why the client is seeking therapy now. Has something happened recently that has made the problem worse? One couple who had been married over 50 years came into therapy, with the wife threatening to leave the marriage and live with one of her daughters. The couple reported the relationship had deteriorated after it was discovered the husband had had an affair nearly 40 years ago. This naturally led the therapist to question why the couple was seeking therapy now. Recent changes in the husband's mood and behavior had further increased the wife's distress, leading her to consider leaving.

We recommend that you ask individuals why they believe the problem exists. This is important for at least two reasons. First, one or more individuals may have good insight as to why the problem or problems exist. When working with couples, for example, you may notice individuals sometimes have good insight into their partner (but often lack insight into their own contribution to the problem). These insights can give you a starting point for hypothesizing, although you will certainly want to entertain other hypotheses. Second, you will need to be careful how you present your interventions, especially if it challenges a client's belief about why a problem exists. Otherwise, you may encounter unexpected resistance. One woman was convinced that her husband had attention-deficit/hyperactivity disorder (ADHD), which she believed explained his behavior. The therapist, however, did not believe the husband had ADHD. The therapist was careful to acknowledge the wife's concern, but he provided psychoeducation on ADHD to support his position that the husband's behavior was better explained by other factors.

ASSESSING CLIENT GOALS

Your initial assessment also includes establishing client goals for therapy. At first blush, these would seem simple enough to define—simply eliminate the presenting problems! A couple, for example, may state that they want to stop fighting. Or parents may want their child to stop acting out.

However, there can be an important difference between eliminating the presenting problem and client goals for therapy. Ideally, you will be able to identify goals that state in positive terms what the clients will be doing rather than what they won't be doing. Charlotte's initially stated goal was to have Brock stop criticizing her all the time. When translated into more positive terms, her goal became "I want Brock to notice and express appreciation for the things I do as a mother and wife."

Assessing client goals can illustrate the principle of "assessment is intervention, and intervention is assessment" stated in the first chapter. It may not be obvious to many clients what they will be doing positively in place of the presenting problem. Thus, even asking this question may begin to get your clients to shift their perspective, creating an early intervention. Some therapists like to borrow from solution-focused therapy and pose the miracle question (de Shazer, 1988), which asks, "Suppose that one night, while you were asleep, there was a miracle and this problem was solved. How would you know? What would be different?"

Ideally, client goals will be compatible when working with a couple or family. However, this is often not the case (Patterson et al., 2009). The therapist may need to reframe or link the family members' goals in a way that makes sense to everyone. A mother may complain about her son's irresponsibility, while the adolescent complains that he does not have enough freedom. The therapist might connect the two concerns by stating the goal is to have the son progress toward becoming an adult. Being an adult is then defined as having both certain responsibilities as well as certain privileges, which go hand in hand.

In couple therapy, each person can have a very different level of commitment to the relationship, which can present special challenges in goal setting. One approach is to initially contract to do a relationship evaluation. Like a house inspection, the evaluation will determine what problems exist, what will be required to fix them, and what is in fine working condition. After the evaluation, each partner can then decide if he or she wants to invest time and effort in repairing the relationship, or move on.

After the relationship evaluation, ideally you will be able to identify goals that will benefit the individual regardless of whether or not the relationship is saved. This can be a particularly effective approach for individuals thinking of leaving the relationship. When Juanita and Harry came to therapy, Harry stated he was very invested in the marriage and would do whatever was necessary to save it. Juanita said that although she still cared for her husband, she did not think that the marriage would work out. She was waiting to leave the marriage until her husband's current health issues were resolved and he was capable of taking care of himself without her aid. However, she was hoping that therapy would make their relationship more peaceful until such time as she could leave. During the relationship evaluation, it became evident that Juanita was reenacting a pattern seen in many of her past intimate relationships. The co-therapists pointed out this pattern and then suggested to Juanita that if she left this marriage and got into another relationship, history was likely to repeat itself. Juanita agreed to examine how this pattern might be changed with the hope that it might improve her marriage, or possibly a future relationship should she decide to end her current marriage.

OTHER EXPECTATIONS FOR THERAPY

Clients bring into the therapy room a variety of other expectations regarding therapy. You should determine whom your client believes should be in therapy, which may need to be negotiated. For example, parents may bring a child into therapy anticipating that you will work with just the child. You may need to educate the parents on the importance of doing family work rather than seeing the child alone. Occasionally an individual will come to therapy with concerns about his or her marriage or relationship and will need encouragement to bring the partner in as well.

Some clients have assumptions regarding how long therapy will last. One client expected therapy to last at least 1 year, and he was surprised when the therapist explained that therapy was typically much briefer at that agency. On the opposite end of the spectrum, some clients expect symptom relief within a session or two, which is often unrealistic.

Clients may also have expectations about the role of the therapist or how therapy will be conducted. Some clients expect their therapist to take a directive, advice-giving role. Other clients see therapy as a place to vent. Clients who have had previous therapy may want or expect you to behave in a manner similar to that of their previous therapists. Therefore, it is wise to ask about previous therapy to see what they liked and disliked about their previous experiences. If a previous therapist assigned homework or suggested outside reading, then your client may expect the same of you.

Finally, clients may have their own theories as to how change should occur. Does your client see insight into one's family of origin as important? Does your client see one person as having the problem? Or, is your client open to seeing it as a relational problem that requires changing how people interact? The client's view of the problem and how it should be changed will influence his or her receptivity to certain types of interventions or approaches.

Client expectations can be uncovered at any point in therapy, but this is most likely to occur in the first session. When describing the therapy process, you should encourage clients to ask questions. Client expectations can often be intuited from the questions they ask. If parents ask whether they need to come to therapy, they may be indirectly telling you they do not see their role as essential to the process. You may also want to directly ask clients about their expectations, particularly if you sense that they may be different from yours.

In some cases, you may discover clients hold very different expectations from you regarding how therapy will be conducted. Some client expectations are rigid and inflexible, while others are flexible and easily negotiated. If a client's expectations are being rigidly held to, you will need to decide if you can operate within these expectations. Mrs. Bryan was concerned about her 21-year-old son who lived with her. He had dropped out of community college and was struggling to find a job. The mother contacted the therapist and asked that her son be seen. She insisted on being informed as to the young man's social activities and alcohol and drug use. The therapist explained the importance of confidentiality in working with the young man, but Mrs. Bryan said that if she paid the bill, then she deserved to have this information. The therapist was unable to comply with her request and made it clear that without confidentiality, he could not do the therapy.

ASSESSING CLIENT MOTIVATION

Clients come into therapy with various levels of motivation. It is important to gauge each client's level of motivation and the factors that affect it. The level of pain or distress that individuals are experiencing often correlates with their level of motivation. Individuals with a high level of emotional pain are generally more motivated to do something different to alleviate their distress. Conversely, individuals who are in little or no emotional pain may have little incentive to change. Robert vented to his therapist each week about his relationship with his father. He was more irritated than distressed and did not seem invested in improving the relationship or looking at his own behaviors that might be contributing to the problems. In one session, the therapist questioned whether Robert was distressed enough by the problem to make the necessary changes to resolve the issue. Robert said he was. However, he returned 2 weeks later to say he had thought about the therapist's words, and he had since concluded that he was not sufficiently bothered by the problem to invest the necessary time and effort to fix it. Therefore, Robert and the therapist agreed to end therapy.

Whether clients enter therapy voluntarily may be another indicator of motivation. Some clients may be court mandated to attend therapy or forced by family members to attend therapy. An adolescent may be told to come to therapy by his or her parents, or a mate may be threatened with divorce if he or she does not agree to therapy. Involuntary clients may not perceive that a problem exists and therefore have little motivation to change. In these situations, one possible approach is to tell the reluctant client that he or she has at least one problem—someone is making them come to therapy! The motivation for therapy at that point can be framed as making the necessary changes so that he or she will no longer be forced to attend therapy.

Depression can also impact a client's motivation for change. The lack of motivation associated with moderate to severe depression can create a significant impediment to therapy. Shirley presented to therapy with severe depression. Initially therapy was unsuccessful in addressing her depression and its underlying causes. Fortunately, Shirley was referred for a medical evaluation early in therapy and was placed on an antidepressant. As her depression began to lift due to her medication, she began making progress in therapy. She began to apply what she was learning in therapy, which addressed the underlying causes of her depression.

Potential negative consequences to change must also be considered when assessing a client's motivation for change. Change is often anxiety producing because clients are unsure of what it will bring. Clients may also have specific fears or concerns regarding change. If you ask them to be vulnerable, will they be rejected or give their partner further ammunition in a later fight? Therefore, you may want to ask your clients if they have any fears about making changes. You can help them determine the extent to which these fears are realistic. In some cases, clients may discover that the potential negative consequences outweigh the potential benefits of change, which will require therapy to move toward fostering acceptance rather than change.

Prochaska, Norcross, and DiClemente (1995) have developed a model that describes the various stages clients proceed through as they attempt to change. In the initial precontemplation stage, individuals are not thinking of changing their behavior. In the subsequent contemplation stage, individuals are thinking about changing their behavior within the next 6 months. This is followed by the preparation stage, where individuals plan to change their behavior within the next month.

In the action stage, individual are actively trying to change their behavior. The last stage, the maintenance stage, is defined as the period 6 months after the action stage begins and continues until the behavior has been changed (e.g., smoking has stopped).

Therapy will need to take into consideration where clients are in this change process. Clients who are in the precontemplative or contemplative stages may not be receptive to direct suggestions for change. Instead, you may want to try motivational interviewing (Miller & Rollnick, 2002), an approach that can be used to explore and strengthen a client's motivation for change. Motivational interviewing uses a directive, client-centered approach to help the client explore and ultimately resolve his or her ambivalence regarding change. This is accomplished by helping the client articulate the factors that both restrain and promote the desire for change. In motivational interviewing, the therapist does not attempt to directly persuade or challenge the client to change, but affirms the client's freedom of choice. The therapist elicits and selectively reinforces statements made by the client that reflect the existence of a problem, a desire to change, and a belief in one's ability to change.

ATTEMPTED SOLUTIONS

We recommend you explore previous solutions the clients have tried. Knowing what the clients have attempted before may prevent you from prematurely offering a similar solution that has already been tried unsuccessfully or rejected, which could undermine your credibility.

When soliciting attempted solutions, it may be important to assess specifically what was tried. A parent may tell you that he or she already tried a behavioral chart, an intervention that you had tentatively thought might be worthwhile. Eliciting specifics will enable you to determine if the parent used the behavioral chart properly or stayed with the intervention for a sufficient length of time.

You should also explore what happened as a result of the attempted solution. In some cases, the attempted solution may have offered a partial relief but was not sufficient to eliminate the problem. On the opposite end, some attempted solutions make the situation worse. This was the case for Henri, a 28-year-old who presented in therapy with concerns about his drinking. Both of his parents are alcoholics, and he was afraid that his drinking was becoming problematic. He had missed a few days of work and was worried about drinking and driving. He had attempted to control his drinking by eliminating any alcohol intake during the weekdays and restricting his drinking to only weekends. This experiment went well for the first 2 weeks, and then he began to notice a change in his drinking on the weekends. He said he found that he anticipated the opportunity to drink so much that it became his primary focus during the week. When the weekend came he drank excessively because, he said, he "felt trapped and wanted to drink all I can, while I can." His attempted solution actually made the problem worse.

You may also want to ask about solutions that others have proposed but the clients did not try. Again, you don't want to propose an idea that the clients have already rejected. If you think it is an idea that has merit, you should carefully inquire as to why the idea was rejected. The answer may give you clues to possible negative consequences that will need to be taken into consideration.

You will also want to know if clients have attempted therapy before to address the problem. To what extent was previous therapy helpful or unsuccessful? If therapy was unsuccessful, then you will want to learn what approach was used so you can try a different approach. In addition, you will want to avoid repeating mistakes made by previous therapists. One couple complained that their previous therapist had recommended the couple split up. Knowing a client's previous history with therapy may also help you to have realistic expectations. One couple reported that they had had therapy with four other therapists in the past year, all of it unsuccessful. Obviously the beginning therapist seeing this couple should not be surprised if therapy ends prematurely before significant change occurs.

CONCERNS ABOUT THERAPY OR THERAPIST COMPETENCE

Concerns about therapy or the therapist are most likely to arise during the initial session. Clients may question, for example, how helpful therapy can be. Some clients hold the belief that therapy is primarily for "crazy people" and may attach a stigma to being in therapy. For these clients, it may be helpful to reframe therapy using a coaching metaphor, noting that even the best athletes benefit from coaching. For others, it may work best to portray therapists as relationship consultants.

Concerns regarding a therapist usually center on youth or inexperience. Clients may question whether a young therapist has the necessary clinical experience to be helpful. They may also question a therapist's credibility if he or she lacks some important life experience, such as being married or having children. Credibility issues can also arise based on a therapist's characteristics, such as gender, race and ethnicity, or sexual orientation. A person of color may question whether a white therapist can truly understand what it means to be part of a minority culture or experience discrimination.

Dealing with issues of credibility can be difficult for beginning therapists, particularly since they often feel insecure about their abilities in the first place (Patterson et al., 2009). If you can respond to your clients' concerns in a nondefensive manner, this may bolster their confidence in you. You need to remember that even beginning therapists have something to offer clients, including compassion and support. Beginning therapists can also offer helpful clinical insights by being an objective third party or by drawing upon their training.

Reasons other than a therapist's experience can be a basis for concern. One female client told her male therapist she was uncomfortable working with him because of molestation by another man. She felt it would be safer for her to explore these issues in therapy if the therapist was a woman. Some clients want a therapist who shares their religious beliefs or convictions.

If concerns are raised in a general or vague manner, you may need to pinpoint what the specific issue or issues are in order to intervene more effectively. A lesbian client named Gwen expressed concerns about working with a "straight" female therapist at the beginning of the initial session. The therapist initially assumed that Gwen's concerns were based on her admitted lack of experience working with gay and lesbian clients. At the end of the session, however, Gwen expressed enthusiasm about continuing her work with the therapist. Upon further inquiry, Gwen explained she had feared the therapist would judge her because of her sexual orientation. However, she found this was not the case and felt very comfortable with the therapist because of her warm and nonjudgmental presence.

IDENTIFYING STRENGTHS AND RESOURCES

An important part of assessment in the initial interview and throughout therapy is the identification of client strengths and resources. Indeed, an effective way to conclude an initial interview is to highlight the clients' strengths. This is reassuring to clients because they often fear you will look unfavorably upon them. It can also foster a sense of hope that things can change, especially if the clients were not consciously aware of these strengths.

Client strengths can exist in a number of areas. First, listen carefully for personal qualities that can be emphasized as strengths. Clients' insights can be validated. An individual's resilience in surviving a traumatic experience can also be highlighted as a strength. In some instances, you may find that an apparent weakness may actually be a positive quality in a different context. Jorge, a 9-year-old boy, talked too much in class and at times spoke up without raising his hand. His comments were sometimes inappropriate and tended to distract the class. Jorge was a gifted athlete who was admired by many of his classmates. On the playground, he showed exceptional athletic ability and leadership qualities. Outside of the classroom setting, he was able to find a more constructive outlet for his very high energy level. Similarly, behaviors that are maladaptive in the present may have been adaptive once in a different context. Susan, who was conflict avoidant with her husband, had learned this pattern of coping in her childhood. To avoid being hit, Susan would hide in her room when her alcoholic father became angry or drunk.

When identifying client strengths, it can be diagnostically helpful to directly ask individuals what strengths they possess. A client who struggles to identify personal strengths may have self-esteem issues. You might also ask individuals to comment on the strengths of other family members. Hearing a partner or family member comment on one's strengths can build a sense of hope and goodwill. Others may note strengths that the individual does not recognize or may be reluctant to state for fear of appearing vain. It is also diagnostic, however, if individuals cannot identify strengths in their partner or other family members. Parents who cannot identify a child's strengths may have become so demoralized by their child's behavior that they overlook his or her positive traits. Encouraging parents to "catch the child doing good" can challenge this deficit-oriented view of their child.

A second area in which to explore client strengths is within relationships. A couple's shared interests might be highlighted, for example, or their ability to enjoy each other's company. Even differences in personality can be labeled as a strength based on their potential to complement one another.

Clients' participation in therapy can be pointed out as a strength. Individuals who seek out therapy preventatively or prior to a crisis can be complimented on their wisdom in seeking out help before things became worse. Clients who are willing to look at their own role in the situation rather than blaming others can be praised. Even clients who reluctantly come to therapy can be applauded for caring enough about the relationship to come despite their reservations.

You should also assess for client resources. While strengths reflect qualities or attitudes that clients possess, we define resources as external factors that can be used by clients for change or to enhance their well-being. Social support is perhaps one of the most important resources for which you should assess. For example, does the individual have family or friends from whom they receive support? Are they able to obtain both emotional and instrumental support from these individuals, or is one or both lacking? Do they belong to a church, community group, or other organization in which they feel a sense of belonging or receive support?

Resources can take other forms. Finances can be an important resource for some clients. Clients with financial resources tend to have more options and opportunities available to them. Some couples have the means to hire a babysitter and spend an evening out on a date, while others cannot afford to do this. Those with more income might also be able to hire a tutor to help a student struggling academically.

CONCLUSION

This chapter has discussed topics that you will want to focus on in the initial interview, with particular emphasis on topics to include in the initial assessment. The areas of assessment addressed in this chapter are applicable across a wide range of clients. Subsequent chapters will focus on how to conduct assessment on specific issues or with different populations. Chapter 4 focuses on how to assess safety issues, including child abuse, suicide, domestic violence, and others. Chapters 5 and 6 focus on assessing adult functioning, including ruling out psychopathology. Chapters 7 and 8 focus on assessment of children and adolescents, with the latter focusing on common disorders within this population.

Chapter 9 discusses how to assess dynamics within a family, while Chapter 10 describes how families need to be assessed within multiple contexts such as transgenerational and life cycle issues. Assessment with couples is examined in Chapters 11 and 12, with the last chapter devoted to special topics within couple therapy (i.e., infidelity, sex, premarital counseling, same-sex couples). Finally, Chapter 13 discusses how to develop a treatment plan using assessment data, as well as how to assess if change is occurring and if clients are ready for termination.

CHAPTER 4

Assessing Issues of Safety

When you made the decision to become a family therapist, your primary passion was likely the idea of helping couples and families improve their relationships. It's unlikely that your career aspirations included working with clients considering suicide, or submitting child abuse reports to child protective services. Such experiences and responsibilities can terrify therapists and even make them question their desire to enter this field. The core mission of a family therapist is addressing relationship health. In some cases, however, attending to relationship health includes exploring the possibility of violence—violence to others and violence to self.

Population-based estimates of violence suggest that some type of violence occurs in approximately 15–20% of families. While spousal abuse and physical abuse of children are probably the most common forms of violence, elder abuse is becoming increasingly common. In this chapter, we discuss the assessment of safety issues, including suicide, harm to others, child abuse, elder and dependent adult abuse, and domestic violence. We do not give an exhaustive review of assessment in each area. Rather, our goal is to provide some basic assessment information to help you identify when these safety issues are present and require your attention.

SUICIDE ASSESSMENT

According to the World Health Organization, suicides have increased by 60% worldwide during the last 45 years, and suicide is among the three leading causes of death among 15- to 44-year-olds (World Health Organization, 2009). Many people attempt suicide but do not ultimately kill themselves, so the rate of suicide attempts is actually much higher. In fact, some mental health experts distinguish between "suicide attempters" who actually plan to die versus sufferers who make suicidal gestures as a means of communicating pain. A key difference between the groups is the lethality of the means. For example, men, especially elderly and young men, are more likely to use lethal means such as guns whereas attempters, often females, are more likely to use means such as pills or cutting. Nevertheless, any suicidal gesture or attempt should be taken seriously.

Several myths might prevent beginning therapists from addressing their clients' suicidal feelings (World Health Organization, 2000). The first myth is that clients who talk about suicide rarely follow through on their ideas. While it is true that most people who have suicidal thoughts will not ultimately take their lives, it is also true that most people who kill themselves have communicated their intent to someone in the weeks and months before they die. Another myth is that asking a client about suicidal thoughts might serve as the impetus for the client's suicide. In fact, asking about suicidal thoughts and feelings can often reduce the sufferer's anxiety and obsessions about death. An empathic understanding of the client's feelings can help *prevent* the client's suicide attempt. Another myth is that a suicidal client will appear despondent and miserable. Often, this is not the case. In fact, some clients who have recently finalized their decision to commit suicide may appear calm and detached. After months of ruminating, they finalize their decision, and they may also decide not to share their plans with anyone. In addition, a client's plan and intent may vary over time depending on his or her circumstances. Therapists should not assume that a client's appearance reflects the risk of suicidal intent.

As a therapist, you can use the known predictors of suicide to assess risk in your clients. Known risk factors include (Nock & Kessler, 2006):

- *Gender.* More females attempt suicide, but males are more likely to actually kill themselves.

- *Age.* Historically elderly men (above 60 years) have been the demographic group most likely to commit suicide. But in recent years, young adults (15–30) have become an equally high-risk group.

• *Marital status.* Divorced, widowed, and single people are at increased risk of suicide. Marriage is more protective for men than women in terms of suicide risk. Loneliness is a risk factor for suicide. Feeling connected to another person protects people from suicidal plans.

• *Mental health problems.* Depression, impulse problems, schizophrenia, and personality disorders such as borderline personality disorder or antisocial personality disorder all put an individual at risk for suicide. Risk is greater for clients with two or more mental disorders.

• *Specific and psychological losses.* Job or personal losses, gambling losses, financial loss, and feelings of humiliation, shame, and hopelessness predispose the person to want to die.

• *Previous attempts.* Previous suicide attempts are one of the strongest predictors of completed suicide, although many individuals attempt suicide only once and are ambivalent about dying even during the first attempt. Further attempts over an extended period predict eventual suicide completion. Talking about suicide or wishing to die, even without a suicide attempt, also predicts a future attempt.

• *Chronic illness or chronic pain.* Unabated pain and illness, especially in the elderly, put the people at risk for suicide.

• *Substance abuse.* Drug and alcohol use often disinhibit people. They lose their ability to think clearly and become more impulsive. Protective barriers such as thoughtful reflection may be lost during substance use. Thus, the person is more likely to spontaneously attempt suicide.

• *Lethality of means.* Having a gun in the house or other potentially lethal circumstances such as living on a high floor in an apartment building or having toxic medications on hand provide means of committing suicide. Many suicidal patients report that they carefully prepare and rehearse their suicide plan for weeks before they actually make an attempt.

• *Trauma in childhood.* Sexual or physical abuse as a child is a risk factor for suicide. Clients who had years of abuse are more at risk than clients who had a one-time event such as a rape or single beating.

• *Completed suicides in the community or family.* Suicides carried out by family, friends, or even acquaintances predict further suicides. Some experts believe that this risk is increased when the media or other authorities glamorize or idealize suicide attempts.

Interviewing a Suicidal Client

If you suspect that your client might be considering suicide, you should ask in detail about his or her plans. But the discussion will be more effective if you have previously established rapport. If you have time, the first step in helping a suicidal client is to communicate your caring, concern, and understanding before you ever broach the subject. Shea (1999) identifies specific skills and techniques that a therapist can use when interviewing a suicidal client. Those skills include:

- *Normalization.* The therapist lets the client know that it is understandable to feel the way he or she does. In essence, the therapist communicates "I understand how difficult your circumstances and feelings are. Other clients have thought about killing themselves in these difficult circumstances. I'm wondering if you have thought of dying or killing yourself?"

- *Gentle assumption.* The therapist asks questions in a way that assumes the client has suicidal thoughts or feelings (as opposed to communicating surprise or worry about the client's suicidal thoughts). For example, the therapist might say, "What ways have you thought about killing yourself?"

- *Behavioral incidents.* The therapist keeps asking for more specific details of the plan including what, when, why, and how. The therapist wants to assess how meticulous the client has been in planning his or her suicide because the level of detail suggests the seriousness of intent. For example, the therapist might say, "You said that you'd want to make sure you died, so you'd take enough of drug X to die. What dose have you thought about taking?"

- *Denial of the specific.* The therapist asks about other ways the client might commit suicide. For example, the therapist might ask, "Have you thought about hanging yourself (taking pills, cutting yourself, jumping off a bridge, etc.)?" The therapist continues asking until the client denies interest in specific means of suicide.

Ensuring the Safety of a Suicidal Client

Using these techniques will help the therapist uncover the extent of the client's planning and actual attempts. At the same time, the therapist must assess the urgency of ensuring that client's safety. If the therapist believes the risk is urgent, several options exist. In general, the client needs to be in a safe place, and often the most expedient way to ensure this is to have someone take the client to the emergency room of a hospital for further evaluation and possible admission. If the therapist believes that the client is at imminent risk, the client cannot be left alone. In our experience, nursing staff or other clinic staff, family members, or friends have been asked to stay with the suicidal client and transport him or her to the emergency room. The therapist notifies the emergency room physician that the client is coming and ensures that the client will not be left alone.

Other more challenging scenarios can also arise. For example, during a phone conversation, a client might report that he is going to kill himself immediately. In this situation, the therapist can call the police and the police will go the client's home. At times, therapists have had to cancel their next appointments so they can stay with their suicidal client until the client's safety is ensured. Also, imminent suicide is a legal justification to both break confidentiality and to have a client hospitalized involuntarily. The underlying principle in all of these difficult scenarios is that the therapist must do everything in his or her power to ensure the client's safety. Usually the clients, who are ambivalent about dying, are appreciative of their therapist's care and concern and will willingly accept the protective measures that therapists suggest.

The therapist should also address the client's suicidal feelings in non-urgent situations. Many therapists will ask clients to sign an agreement that the client and therapist create together, documenting the client's commitment to take the necessary steps for safety if he or she is feeling suicidal. Other options include bringing family members into the discussion and reducing any feelings of secrecy, shame, or isolation that suicidal clients feel by encouraging them to openly share their feelings.

ASSESSING HARM TO OTHERS

In addition to your responsibility to protect clients from self-harm, you also have a duty to protect individuals who are threatened by your clients. Because threats to others can sometimes be vague and unclear, it can be helpful to consider several factors in your assessment of threats to others. Borum and Reddy (2001) have suggested six factors that therapists can use, which together form the acronym ACTION:

- Attitudes (attitudes that support or facilitate violence)—Does the client believe that violence is justified in certain situations?
- Capacity—Does the client have access to the means (e.g., weapons) to carry out threats?
- Thresholds crossed—Does the client have a plan, and what is the extent to which he or she has begun to put a plan into action?
- Intent—Does a client's comment reveal serious intent to harm others, or is it a general comment that reflects frustration but no serious intent to harm another person?
- Others' reactions and responses—Have others encouraged or discouraged the individual's hostile behavior?
- Noncompliance with risk reduction—Does the client show an unwillingness to consider alternatives to harming others?

You should also consider other risk factors, such as a history of violence toward others. Has the client used violence toward others in the past or carried through on previous threats? You should also explore whether the individual has a history of mental instability or drug/alcohol abuse that may predispose him or her to violence.

The nature and seriousness of the threat will determine what steps are necessary to protect others from harm. For example, you may need to seek hospitalization for a client if he or she poses a serious threat to others. In some cases, your duty to protect may result in needing to notify the intended victims of potential harm. This "duty to warn" dates back to the 1970s: Tatiana Tarasoff, a student at the University of California, Berkeley, was killed by a man who reported to his psychologist that he intended to kill her. Neither Tatiana nor her parents received any warning of the client's threat. The California Supreme Court (*Tarasoff v. Regents of the University of California*) ruled the following:

> When a therapist determines that his patient presents a serious danger of violence to another, he incurs an obligation to use reasonable care to protect the intended victim against such danger. The discharge of this duty may call for the therapist to warn the intended victim or to take whatever other steps are reasonably necessary under the circumstances.

Therapists should be aware of their state laws regarding duty to warn issues. You may need to consider several elements in evaluating whether a duty to warn exists. In California, for example, therapists must determine the following[1]:

• *Who is making the threat?* Your client must be the person who is threatening harm to someone. If a client tells you that his friend is going to kill someone, there is no duty to warn (and you may be guilty of a breach of confidentiality if you warn).

• *How did you learn of the threat?* A duty to warn exists if the client reports directly to you a threat. As a result of *Ewing v. Goldstein* and *Ewing v. Northridge Hospital Medical Center*, the duty to warn was expanded to include credible warnings about a client's threatened violence from the client's immediate family members.

• *Is there a serious and/or imminent danger of physical violence?* Is there a threat of physical violence to a person (bodily harm, not only murder)? Is the threat deemed serious and imminent based on the risk factors discussed earlier (e.g., ACTION, history of violence)?

• *Is there an identifiable victim?* The threat must be toward someone who is readily identifiable. You are obligated to take reasonable steps to identify potential victims (e.g., if the patient says "I am going to kill her," you must inquire as to who the victim is). You do not need to become a private investigator, but you need to inquire about potential victims.

CHILD ABUSE

In addition to developing a safe environment and listening to their experiences and concerns, we are obligated to find out if children who become our clients are victims of child abuse. Child abuse, which can be committed by any person, regardless of age or relationship to the child, can occur in a variety of ways:

• *Physical abuse.* Physical abuse is physical injury that is inflicted by other than accidental means (e.g., intentional) on a child by another person. This does not include a mutual scuffle between minors or reasonable parental discipline.

---

[1] All laws described in this chapter come from our home state of California. Please check the laws in your state to see how they are similar to or different from California law.

- *Neglect.* There are two types: (1) severe, such as malnutrition, and (2) general, when a child is not provided with adequate food, clothing, shelter, medical care, or supervision, which includes children who have run away.

- *Sexual abuse.* Includes both sexual acts without consent (e.g., rape, sodomy, incest, masturbating in front of a child) and sexual acts with consent, depending upon the age of the two parties. For example, in California, consensual sex between a minor and another person is reportable if any of the following conditions is met: (1) child under 14 and perpetrator 14 or over, (2) child under 16 and perpetrator 21 or over, or (3) child 14 or 15 and perpetrator 10 years or more older.

- *Emotional abuse.* Although difficult to define, emotional abuse can arise when a child is exposed to behavior that is psychologically harmful. Psychological harm can occur in a number of different ways, including being insulted or called names, being bullied or threatened, being a victim of other forms of abuse, or witnessing violence against others (e.g., domestic violence). Emotional abuse may also arise through neglect.

Of the three million children who are abused each year, neglect and physical abuse account for the largest majority of reports to child protective services (Ketring, 2007). While girls are much more likely than boys to be sexually abused, boys are more likely to be physically abused and neglected (Sedlack & Broadhurst, 1996). Because many clients will not self-report abuse and/or don't recognize that their actions or the actions of others are abusive, it's incumbent upon you to regularly screen clients for child abuse and identify risk factors for abuse.

Physical abuse should be suspected if children give evasive answers or unconvincing stories as to how they obtained their injuries (e.g., bruises, burns, welts, broken bones). Adult characteristics that may increase the likelihood of child abuse include depression, substance abuse, a history of abuse, and domestic violence (Ketring, 2007; Wolff, 1999). When asked about how they discipline their children, parents may disclose examples that qualify as physical abuse, even though they may feel their actions are justified (e.g., "The belt against his backside is the only way to get him to listen").

Like physical abuse, sexual abuse occurs more frequently than reported. Detection is often left to the therapist. If a child indicates several of the following symptoms, further interviewing needs to be done:

1. Physically, a child may display sleep disturbances, encopresis or enuresis, complain of abdominal pain, or suffer from appetite disturbances with corresponding weight change.
2. Behaviorally, a child may manifest a sudden unexplained change in behavior (anxiety or depression), regressive behavior, or overly sexualized behavior or knowledge given the child's age, experience suicidal thoughts, run away, or abuse substances
3. Socially, family conditions may include a child's parentified role, inadequate parental coping skills, marital difficulties leading to one parent seeking physical affection from the child, isolated social context, alcohol or drug use, and a history of parental sexual abuse (Edwards & Gil, 1986).

Assessing for child abuse goes beyond just determining what type of abuse, if any, a child has suffered and reporting the abuse to child protective services. If a child has been abused, you will also want to explore the extent to which a child or adolescent has developed trauma-related symptoms, which can arise due to several interacting variables (Gil, 2006): (1) predisposing factors, such as the quality of parent–child attachments and amount of personal resources; (2) characteristics of the trauma, including the type, number of times, and age of exposure to abuse; and (3) posttrauma variables, such as amount and type of social support.

DEPENDENT AND ELDER ABUSE

As the baby boomer generation transitions into older adulthood and longevity continues to increase, adult children will increasingly be put in the position of caring for their aging parents, and family therapists will increasingly be confronted with presenting problems associated with family caregiving. Just as you assess children and their family members for possible child abuse, you also need to assess for possible dependent adult and elder abuse. In California, elders are defined as anyone 65 and older. Dependent adults are between the ages of 18 and 64 and have physical or mental limitations that restrict their ability to carry out normal activities or to protect their own rights. Elder and dependent abuse can take many forms, including:

- Physical abuse
- Sexual abuse

- Neglect
- Financial abuse
- Abandonment
- Isolation
- Abduction
- Emotional abuse

As with child abuse, the dependent adult or elder may not report or recognize abuse. In addition to asking about unexplained bruises or marks, you will want to ask caretakers about how they manage the elder or dependent individual, particularly when the caretaker feels burned out and frustrated. Possible signs of neglect include the individual not being properly groomed, or not receiving appropriate care for medical or physical needs. As with child abuse, knowledge or reasonable suspicion of elder or dependent abuse may require a mandated report to adult protective services (or other appropriate authorities depending upon state law).

DOMESTIC VIOLENCE

Individuals working with couples need to be vigilant about the possibility of domestic or intimate partner violence. It is estimated that each year intimate partner violence results in two million injuries to women over the age of 18, with over a quarter of them requiring medical attention (National Center for Injury Prevention and Control, 2003). Individuals who experience domestic violence can also suffer serious psychological consequences. The impact of domestic violence can extend beyond the couple, and can significantly affect children who witness it. Despite the importance and prevalence of domestic violence, many clinicians fail to properly assess for it (Schacht, Dimidjian, George, & Berns, 2009).

Therefore, we recommend you routinely evaluate all couples for domestic violence (Bograd & Mederos, 1999; Holtzworth-Munroe, Clements, & Farris, 2005; Riggs, Caulfield, & Street, 2000). When assessing how couples handle conflict, you can ask them to describe what an argument or fight looks like. Some couples will divulge at this point that they get physical with one another. If not, it is good to ask a follow-up question such as "Have your arguments ever gotten to the point where one or both of you became physical with the other?" By asking the question in this way, you encourage the couple to admit to other behaviors beyond just hitting, which may include pushing or shoving one's partner, or restraining the partner from leaving. The couple may be more willing to disclose incidences if the question is framed as inquiring about the past rather than asking if the behaviors are current. If the couple admits to any incidences in the past, it is obviously important to follow up and inquire as to when the most recent incident occurred. The risk of domestic violence occurring in the future is higher the more recent the last incidence.

Some individuals will deny any domestic violence during a conjoint session for fear a disclosure of this nature will lead to violence at home after the session. As a result, some clients will not admit to any domestic violence unless asked privately in an individual session. For this reason, many clinicians recommend that you have at least one individual session with each partner to rule out domestic violence (e.g., Bograd & Mederos, 1999; Stith, Rosen, & McCollum, 2003), often with the stated purpose of conducting an individual history. A clinician would also be wise to consider the possibility of domestic violence if one partner (particularly the male) expresses strong reservations about individual sessions, which may be an attempt to prevent the disclosure of the problem.

Domestic violence may be uncovered in other ways. You should suspect domestic violence if an individual has sustained injuries and does not offer a plausible explanation for them. Individuals who appear fearful or reticent about answering questions in conjoint sessions should raise suspicion. Assessment measures can sometimes provide evidence of domestic violence. The Conflict Tactics Scale (Straus, 1979) and the Revised Conflict Tactics Scale (Straus, Hamby, Boney-McCoy, & Sugarman, 1996) are frequently used to screen for domestic violence. You should also pay attention to your own internal responses, such as a concern for a family member's safety, or perhaps your own sense of fearfulness, intimidation, or concern for personal safety.

If you uncover domestic violence, it will be important to determine the type, particularly since this will have implications as to the type of treatment that is most appropriate (Greene & Bogo, 2002; Holtzworth-Munroe, Clements, & Farris, 2005). The first type is sometimes referred to as battering or patriarchal terrorism. In this type of violence, the perpetrator uses violence to exert control over the partner. Typically men are the perpetrator in this type of violence. Perpetrators who commit battering or patriarchal terrorism may be of two subtypes, violent/antisocial men or borderline/dysphoric men. Conjoint couple therapy would be contraindicated for this type of domestic violence.

In the second type of violence, partners intermittently become physical with one another when arguments escalate. This has sometimes been called common couple violence. In contrast to patriarchal terrorism, the perpetrator does not use violence as a pervasive pattern of control. Unlike patriarchal terrorism, which is typically male-to-female violence, either the man or the woman may initiate the violence. Although common couple violence typically involves less severe acts of aggression, the risk for physical and emotion harm still exists. Regardless of the type, you need to take the violence seriously and insist that it stop.

Conjoint couple therapy may be feasible for couples struggling with common couple violence, but not for battering or patriarchal terrorism. Therefore, distinguishing between the two types is important. According to Greene and Bogo (2002), clinicians can use four factors to make this distinction. First, you should assess if the perpetrator uses a variety of control tactics besides violence, which is often evident in patriarchal terrorism but not in common couple violence. These control tactics may include emotional abuse, isolation, threats, and control of finances or other resources. Second, you should determine the motivation behind the violence. In patriarchal terrorism, the perpetrator's goal is to establish control over his partner, which is generally not true in common couple violence. Third, you need to assess the impact of the violence on victim. The impact of violence is usually more severe for victims of patriarchal terrorism because the type of violence used is often more severe. Physical and emotional well-being, occupational functioning, and relationships with those outside the couple (e.g., friends, family) are more likely to be impacted for victims of patriarchal terrorism. Finally, the individual's subjective experience of the violence should be assessed. In common couple violence, individuals may not fear their partner, whereas individuals typically fear their partner in patriarchal terrorism.

Holtzworth-Munroe et al. (2005) suggest several conditions must be met before it is safe to do conjoint work. They state that conjoint work is only appropriate for low to moderate levels of aggression when there is no imminent risk of physical harm. In addition, individuals must not fear their partner, or feel they cannot be honest in therapy. Finally, both parties must want the relationship to continue, and be willing acknowledge that any form of violence is problematic and needs to stop.

You should do a careful history/assessment for substance abuse in couples, particularly those with any history of domestic violence. Alcohol or drug use can lower inhibitions, resulting in a significantly higher risk of violence. In some cases, reduction or elimination of substance use may be required to successfully to prevent further violence.

Safety plan

K

When domestic violence is a concern, assess whether the individuals have a safety plan in place. If not, then this should be a treatment priority. When assessing an individual's safety plan, ask if she has someone she can go to if she feels unsafe, such as a friend or family member. If not, brainstorm options, including giving information on domestic violence shelters. Does the client have a means for leaving, such as a car? Does she have a spare key to the car if she is concerned about her partner trying to prevent her from leaving? You should also inquire if she has access to emergency funds. The individual should have easy access to money, credit cards, or other important documents should she need to leave quickly.

You also need to assess whether children have witnessed any domestic violence. If so, were they ever in danger of being physically hurt? Some children may try to protect a parent by intervening or getting between the two adults. Even if children are not at risk for physical harm, they may experience emotional harm from witnessing domestic violence. Therefore, you should attempt to assess what the children observed and its potential impact on them. If children witnessed domestic violence, you may need to make a child abuse report with the proper authorities. In California, for example, therapists would be mandated to make a report if children were at risk for physical harm due to domestic violence. MFTs in California are permitted (but not required) to make a child abuse report if they believe the child experienced emotional abuse by witnessing the violence.

CONCLUSION

In this chapter, we've explored a range of issues that help shape our legal and ethical responsibilities as mental health professionals. Although assessment of these issues can be uncomfortable for therapists and clients, an essential part of our role as family therapists is to care for the well-being of our clients and of individuals in relationships with them. At times, therapists can view the assessment of danger as "playing investigator," and they worry that such queries and possible actions will damage their therapeutic relationship with a client. Although it's certainly possible, in most cases we've found that therapists feel a sense of relief when they identify a problem and, if needed, take action to protect someone.

CHAPTER 5

Assessing Health and Well-Being in Adults

BEYOND DSM DIAGNOSIS

The historical influence of the medical model encourages therapists to obtain a list of symptoms from their clients. Many therapists today are trained to conduct standardized, structured assessment interviews that will guide them to their patients' diagnoses, and the *Diagnostic and Statistical Manual of Mental Disorder* (DSM), which is published by the American Psychiatric Association, often serves as their primary reference. The DSM was originally developed by American military health professionals between the 1920s and the 1940s. Since then, it has been revised every few years to include updates and changes based on recent research. The editors of the DSM aspire to provide a comprehensive, scientific manual that describes individual mental health disorders. However, most clinicians believe that clients' assessments should involve more than a DSM list of symptoms. In fact, the editors of the DSM created the multiaxial evaluation system (described in the next chapter) to provide a more comprehensive picture of clients.

In recent years, other influences have begun to shape clinical assessment in new and exciting ways. Positive psychology has changed the assessment focus to questions about happiness instead of psychopathology. Instead of asking, "What makes clients sick?" positive psychology asks, "What makes clients happy?" "What are the markers of an emotionally healthy life and a life well lived?" Also, neuroscientists and stress researchers have raised questions about how clients respond to stress and how the brain is affected by stress. In addition, social and developmental psychologists have posited the critical role of emotional process both in attachment bonds and in social interaction. Finally, Eastern thought, particularly in the form of Buddhist tenets, has influenced Western psychology (Kornfield, 2009). Instead of focusing on change in therapy, therapists have begun to embrace helping clients move toward "acceptance and commitment." For example, marital therapists might help couples accept each other's vulnerabilities and human foibles instead of trying to change each other (Harris, 2009).

When you are conducting an assessment, we hope you will consider the new information about human development and happiness. We suggest that you conduct a comprehensive, biopsychosocial-systems assessment of your client. Payers, employers, government regulators, and other authorities will require that you obtain specific information related to diagnosis. In this chapter, we provide suggestions for assessments that extend beyond traditional, medical-model assessment and provide a more complete picture of an adult.

STRESS AND COPING

Most people feel some reluctance to seek help from mental health professionals. Even now, stigma, cost, hopelessness, and a host of other factors prevent people from starting therapy. In fact, people often live with problems and pain for many years before they ever enter the therapist's office. Thus, when clients finally seek therapy, they are often motivated by significant pain or fear.

A helpful body of literature for understanding clients' struggles is the research on stress and coping. Many people initially seek therapy because of new life stressors, and they hope that the therapist can help them identify ways of coping. In fact, Axis IV of the DSM expands the range of stressors clients face that can be assessed. Also, the DSM distinguishes between stressors with the following diagnoses: adjustment disorders, acute stress disorder, and posttraumatic stress disorder. The severity of the event, the intensity of the client's response to the event, and the length of time the symptoms last vary among these diagnoses. Usually, a client faces more than one challenge. If you are not an expert on the effects of chronic lifestyle stressors such as migration or poverty, you may inadvertently ignore their impact and focus instead on acute events. When conducting an assessment, consider all possible stressors.

Stress has several components (Kamarck & Anderson, 2006). In general, stress includes events that require a response or change, the client's evaluation of his or her ability to adequately respond to the event, and the client's actual response. Stressors include both short-term stress (getting divorced) and longer-term stress (not having enough money to live on after the divorce). In addition, Sapolsky (1998) points out that humans have a unique source of stress—their brains. He suggests that humans, unlike primates, can get stressed simply by thinking and that constant stressful thoughts can make us ill. In fact, recent research on depression suggests that our stress response, specifically the release of a type of hormone called glucocorticoids, can trigger clinical depression. Stress also affects our physical health including cardiovascular illness, diabetes, sexual dysfunction, immune functioning, sleep, pain, and other areas.

Identifying Stressors

In addition to listening for symptoms that may lead to a clinical diagnosis, we suggest that you listen for stressors as clients tell their stories. List them on the intake as you listen. You may eventually categorize them for the client. For example, you could categorize stressors by control. What can the client control (exercise, seeking family support, getting more information about the problem)? What cannot be changed (the pending death of one's spouse, the loss of a job)? You could also categorize them into acute or chronic categories.

Self-report instruments can also help clients identify stressors. Three possible scales include the Perceived Stress Scale (PSS; Cohen, Kamarck, & Mermelstein, 1983), the Life Experience Survey (LES; Sarason, Johnson, & Siegel, 1978), and the Schedule of Recent Experiences (Holmes & Rahe, 1967). These scales include items such as changes in the number of family get-togethers and major changes in living conditions (building a new home, remodeling, deterioration of home or neighborhood).

Self-report instruments identify only the events, not the client's coping style or behavioral responses to the events. Also, these instruments have the usual weaknesses of self-report instruments, such as dependence on the client's accurate recall of events. But, they also have the strengths of self-report instruments: they are easy to administer, easy to score, and inexpensive. Thus, they are a good starting place for a clinical interview.

Different Types of Stress

The stress literature makes a distinction between normal stress (the birth of a baby) and acute catastrophic stress (a rape). In addition, it examines the effects of environmental stressors like poverty, war, natural disasters, and forced migration. Often, your clients face challenges from all three categories.

Family members also face normal developmental stressors such as getting married, becoming a parent, or facing retirement. Families may be reluctant to admit that they are distressed by these transitions because they feel "everyone goes through this." One way you can help clients is to acknowledge the impact of the event. For example, all parents will remember the physical exhaustion and changes in their marriage when a child was born. Even when families welcome changes, the transition and impact on family relationships can be profound.

Impact of Stress

Physicians discuss *premorbid functioning* when they describe their patients' current illnesses. In essence, premorbid functioning raises the question "How was the client doing before the illness or event?" We recommend that your assessment of clients, regardless of the presenting problems, consider their premorbid functioning. For example, you can easily note physical changes in your client. Clients often report changes including:

- Changes in sleep
- Changes in weight and eating
- Changes in cognitive functioning (memory and executive functioning)
- Changes in libido and sexual behavior
- Changes in physical activity and exercise
- Changes in health-risk behaviors such as drug use or smoking.

Assessment in each of these areas of functioning will be discussed in more detail later in the chapter. However, significant changes in any of the areas above should alert you to look for new events or stressors in the individual's life.

As you listen to your client describe these physical changes, it can sometimes get confusing. The therapist has to determine whether the physical changes are symptoms of other disorders or independent changes. In addition, they may be symptoms of physical disorders beyond the scope of a therapist's practice. For example, head trauma often results in both physical and psychological changes, and clients may be slow to recognize the source of their discomfort. We discuss this further in chapter 6 under the comorbidity. However, often the exact relationship between physical changes and other problems is not totally clear. We recommend that you send your client to a physician if you have concerns. It may be helpful to contact the physician ahead of time and let him or her know your specific questions and concerns.[1]

Coping with Stress

Clients' abilities to cope with stress are influenced by (1) whether they have outlets for fear and frustration, (2) social support, (3) predictability, (4) a sense of control, and (5) a perception of things worsening (Sapolsky, 1998). Each of these elements can be important to assess. Many clients come to therapy to obtain help in both understanding the stressors they face and finding effective responses. Underlying many specific questions in therapy, clients wonder, "What is at stake in this situation?"; "Can I cope?"; "What resources can you provide to help me deal with this situation?"

Ideally, family members help each other through stressful times. As a family therapist, you may wonder aloud about how your client's family relationships, both currently and in the past, should affect your assessment. Siegel (1999) and Keltner (2009) have identified the impact of early relationships and emotional responses that can either benefit or harm clients as they face the tumultuous challenges of life. Often, family members' responses to stress can make the situation worse. For example, a father who starts drinking after he is laid off from work compounds the economic stress that he and his family face. Thus, one

---

[1] We share sample referral letters in our book (Patterson, Albala, McCahill, & Edwards, 2006) *The Therapist's Guide to Psychopharmacology: Working with Patients, Families and Physicians to Optimize Care.*

can consider individual stressors and stressors that affect the entire family.

Case Example of Karen

Karen, age 45, wondered how much longer she could continue juggling the demands of her life. Her sense of responsibility for her two girls, especially since her divorce and subsequent income loss, overwhelmed her. While she would not admit it publicly, she resented the school calling and asking her to do more to help her younger daughter, who was failing math. She could not take on one more responsibility. In addition, she knew that her company had not been profitable for several quarters, and based on seniority, she would be one of the first employees laid off. In addition, her elderly parents depended on her because her siblings lived in different states, and while her mother's health rapidly deteriorated, her father grew increasingly dependent on Karen. Finally, Karen's best friend since childhood had recently died of breast cancer. Karen did not think she had time for "counseling." She was focused on surviving.

Karen had few outlets for her fear and frustration. She did not believe she had control of her life, especially her employment, and she feared that her situation would only worsen. Karen's sister, who lived in another state, begged her to see a therapist for one session to see if it might help. During Karen's initial session, the therapist made some lists:

Chronic stressors

Reduced income due to divorce
Fear of unemployment
Worries about daughters and school failure
Father's increasing dependence

Acute stressors

Mother's decline and anticipated death
Death of best friend

Having the opportunity to talk about her life and identifying the multitude of stressors that she faced was a first step in creating a plan to help Karen cope.

ASSESSING PHYSICAL
WELL-BEING IN ADULTS

Why should a therapist assess an individual's physical well-being? The answer is that physical and psychological well-being are often related. Psychological problems may manifest as physical symptoms. Therefore, assessing physical well-being may provide important clues to psychological disorders. Conversely, physical problems can significantly impact the course of psychological disorders. Poor sleep regulation, for example, can affect the moods of an individual with bipolar disorder. Difficulties in physical well-being can also have an impact on relationships. Insomnia can create irritability, which can intrude on a couple's relationship. Partners may also have significant concerns about each other's health behaviors (e.g., smoking), creating conflict in the relationship.

Sleep

The most common sleep disorder is insomnia, the inability to obtain sleep of adequate length and quality. Some common reasons for insomnia include poor sleep hygiene, restless leg syndrome, stress, menopausal changes, aging, medical conditions, and medication use (Attarian, 2000). Taking a careful sleep history and asking the client to keep a sleep log are two ways to learn more about sleep problems. In the sleep log, the patient records his bedtime, times and durations of awakenings, final awakenings, and naps. You will also want to ask questions about a client's substance use including alcohol and caffeine. Sometimes the client can make small changes such as eliminating naps or reducing caffeine. However, if the sleep problems persist, consider referring your client to a physician. To evaluate sleep hygiene, consider asking questions about:

- Time in bed and activities done in bed
- Exercise and aerobic fitness
- Use of clocks in the bedroom
- Sleep distractions such as partner's snoring or television noise
- Caffeine, alcohol, and narcotics intake
- Routine sleep–wake schedule including naps
- Exposure to early-morning light

In general, beds should be used only for sleeping and sex. Distractions should be minimized. Substance use and activity should be minimized in the hours before sleeping. Having a routine sleep schedule that also involves direct exposure to early-morning light facilitates sleep.

Eating and Weight

Like sleep problems, changes in eating and weight can have many etiologies. The changes may be a symptom of a more significant problem, or eating changes themselves may be the targeted problem. Thus, diet and nutrition are crucial components to integrate into family therapy practice (Edwards, 2002). For example, weight change is often a symptom of depression. It could also be a symptom of a serious illness such as cancer. Dramatic weight changes can also point to eating disorders as the primary diagnosis. One simple way of assessing for weight problems is asking the client to keep track of his or her weight and eating and report any dramatic changes in therapy. Clients can record a baseline weight and also keep a log of their daily eating habits.

Clients can use some excellent websites to assess their weight and eating. For example, they can calculate their body mass index, an indicator of unhealthy weight, by going to *www.nhlbisupport.com/bmi* or *www.cdc.gov/healthyweight/assessing/bmi*. For assessment of their eating habits, including what they eat, clients can go to *www.thenutritionsource. org*, which also provides education about healthy eating. If you have additional concerns about your client's eating and weight, consider a referral to an eating disorders clinic or specialist.

Cognitive Changes

Cognitive changes will become increasingly important to assess as the U.S. population ages. In particular, therapists should pay attention to changes in memory and executive functioning. Memory is often divided into short-term, long-term, and working memory, which is the ability to recall and use multiple facts simultaneously. In general, initial changes happen in short-term memory.

Clients are no longer able to retain and recall recently learned information or experiences. Changes in memory are a natural part of aging and not always a cause for alarm. Nevertheless, in a comprehensive assessment, a therapist should consider any changes in memory especially as the population ages and dementia becomes more common.

An easy way to assess for memory loss is to use the mental status exam described in Chapter 6.

Executive functioning refers to the abilities to organize information, shift attention, sequence tasks in order, anticipate outcomes, and consider multiple solutions to a problem. One way to think about executive functioning is to think about the skills a good executive secretary needs. Executive functioning changes can be symptoms of specific disorders (amnestic disorder, delirium) or symptoms of stress, aging, or chronic illness. For example, deficits in executive functioning have been associated with obesity, diabetes, hypertension, and vascular disease.

Many health-related behaviors—including weight loss, abstinence from substance use, exercise, and adherence to medical regimens—depend on the client's executive functioning skills (Williams & Thayer, 2009). Often, so do treatment interventions. For example, the capacity to carry out the therapist's instructions or the ability to reframe a difficult situation depends on the client's skills. Thus, using the mental status exam as a brief screening tool helps a therapist consider the client's cognitive abilities and also decide if the client needs further evaluation by a physician or neuropsychologist.

Libido and Sexual Behavior

Often clients will not mention concerns about their sexual health even if they are worried. They may be embarrassed, not consider sexuality a domain of therapeutic conversation, or be more concerned about other problems they face. Like the other physical changes mentioned in this section, sexual changes can be a symptom of a larger concern—either mental or physical. The DSM describes specific sexual disorders such as sexual aversion disorder or hypoactive sexual desire disorder.

Often, changes in sexual desire or behavior are related to other struggles, such as depression, exhaustion, or aging. Since sexual behavior is often considered a private matter for clients, therapists should have rapport with their clients and request permission to ask personal questions about sexuality before they begin a sexual assessment. In addition, therapists must communicate comfort and ease with the subject matter while they ask questions. Since clients have varied sexual orientations, the therapist should not assume the sexual orientation of his client. Therapists can ask questions in a way that normalizes the process of seeking a sexual history. For example, a therapist might say, "Many people with depression experience a change in libido. Have you ... ?" The therapist may also inquire as to the client's expectations about therapeutic interventions for sexual concerns.

Content areas that might be explored in a sexual assessment include:

- Currently sexually active?
- Gender preference of sexual partner
- Contraceptive use
- Sexual activities and preferences
- Sexual functioning, including concerns
- Sexually transmitted diseases, including HIV
- Sexual pressure from others, including rape or sexual violence (Rahimian, Bergman, Brown, & Ceniceros, 2006).

Additional information on dealing with sexual issues is provided in chapter 12 on special topics in couple assessment. Sex therapists and physicians can often address concerns that are beyond the therapist's skills or scope of practice. A personal referral with follow-up can ease any awkwardness the client might feel in seeking professional help for sexual concerns.

Physical Activity and Exercise

Health psychologists have identified a miracle treatment for physical pain and mental decline. This treatment protects against aging and partially treats disorders like ADHD and depression. Unlike psychotropic medications, this treatment has no negative side effects and costs nothing, and no prescription is necessary to obtain it. The treatment is physical exercise.

Proven benefits of physical exercise include the following:

- Physical exercise improves clients' moods.
- It reduces the risk of chronic diseases like diabetes or high blood pressure.
- Physical activity promotes better sleep, prevents weight gain, and can facilitate sexual desire.

There are four parts to fitness: aerobic fitness, muscular fitness, stretching, and core stability. However, for a lot of clients, it's best not to suggest they undertake a comprehensive fitness program. Instead, have them aim for small changes, as they can result in significant benefits. The American Heart Association recommends at least 30 minutes of brisk walking or swimming 5 days a week, or 20 minutes of running 3 days a week, plus strength training twice a week. However, even these guidelines may be overwhelming to your depressed client.

Thus, we recommend that you gently inquire about your clients' current exercise regimen. You may also ask about their past physical activity history. Was there a time when your clients felt like they were getting adequate exercise? What was different about that time period? Could they make small changes now to move slightly toward their ideal standard of exercise?

Personal motivation and the belief that change is possible will influence your clients' success. Helping your clients obtain more information about the benefits of exercise, such as the Mayo Clinic's website on fitness (*www.mayoclinic.com/health/fitness/my00396*), can motivate them to make changes. Your inquiry and encouragement regarding the benefits of exercise may be enough to prompt changes in your clients' physical activities.

Health-Risk Behaviors (Smoking)

In Chapter 6, we recommend that you ask about illegal drug use and alcohol use as a routine part of your assessment. In addition, we recommend that you ask about smoking. Your intake form can simply include one or two screening questions about smoking. Information that you might want to obtain includes: current smoking habits including number of cigarettes smoked per day; age that your client started smoking; attempts to quit; and views about the relationship between smoking and his or her mental health struggles. For example, anxious clients often turn to cigarettes to soothe themselves. You might also ask your clients if they want to change their smoking habits as part of their overall changes during therapy. If they answer yes, you may consider referring them to their primary care doctor or another source for smoking cessation.

Case Example of Karen, Continued

Since Karen's divorce, her health habits had changed. She had gained 20 pounds in the first 2 years after her divorce. She had started smoking again, a habit she had proudly given up in her late 20s. Finally, she had given up exercising because she felt like she had no time to exercise, and she had started staying up until 1 or 2 in the morning, even when she had to be at work at 8 the next day. To distract herself from ruminating on her many worries each night, she chose instead to watch late-night television until she fell asleep on the couch.

During the first session, Karen and the therapist also made a list of physical changes she would *eventually* like to make. The therapist also asked Karen to identify which changes she would like to make first and how motivated she was to begin making these changes, all the while emphasizing that Karen would make these decisions, not the therapist. Here is a list of Karen's physical concerns:

- Lose weight (start this summer when it is easier to walk)
- Stop smoking (go see my doctor soon to talk about ways to stop smoking)
- Sleep better (talk to my doctor about ways to improve my sleep)

Karen and the therapist agreed that the next step was to make an appointment with her physician. The therapist said she would call Karen's doctor before the appointment to talk about their shared goals.

ASSESSING PSYCHOSOCIAL WELL-BEING IN ADULTS

Research suggests that several risk and protective factors can affect clients' well-being. These can include personal attributes such as anger or positive outlook. Research also indicates that relationships, both positive and negative, strongly affect clients' happiness.

Living life means facing both positive and negative experiences. In view of that, a simple goal of therapy might be to increase the positive and decrease the negative. In fact, research on individual mental health suggests that a 3 to 1 ratio of positive to negative experiences predicts well-being and a 5 to 1 positive to negative ratio predicts relationship happiness (Fredrickson, 2009; Gottman, 1994). Thus, a simple assessment exercise is for you to help your clients evaluate their positive to negative ratio.

Anger and Hostility

The impact of anger, conflict, and hostility on health and well-being has been examined in recent years. The experience of anger and conflict is an inevitable part of life. In fact, Gottman suggests that anger can be a useful indicator that some situation or interaction needs attention, (Gottman, 1994). However, when brooding anger transforms into contempt, disgust, and hostility, anger can be corrosive both to an individual's health and to his or her relationships. In fact, brooding hostility has been implicated as a source of many negative health outcomes, in particular heart disease, cancer, and infectious diseases.

While expression of anger in relationships carries its own risks, suppressed anger has also been implicated as having damaging effects on mental and physical health. In family literature, expressed emotion, the ongoing expression of resentment and contempt in families, has been implicated as worsening illnesses such as schizophrenia and bipolar disorder (Hooley, 2007). Listen carefully for how your clients approach the inevitable disappointments and resentments of life.

Other Negative Emotions

Powerful negative emotions have also been associated with poor mental and physical health outcomes. Ongoing feelings of shame and humiliation, betrayal, guilt, boredom, suspicion, resentment, and other negative emotions can overwhelm clients and create a downward spiral or what Gottman (1994) calls an absorbing state. In addition, as mentioned earlier in the section on stress, feelings of hopelessness and lack of control over one's circumstances can have damaging effects. Clients begin to view every experience through a prism of negativity. Listen carefully for negative emotions as your client describes her problems and concerns. In addition to addressing the problem situation, therapy might also focus on new, less corrosive ways of viewing the client's life circumstances.

Positive Traits and Emotions that Predict Happiness

Positive psychology has brought a new focus in mental health on why people prosper. Several self-assessment instruments compiled at the University of Pennsylvania can be found at *www.authentichappiness. sas.upenn.edu*. These instruments assess emotions, personal strengths, character strengths, sense of purpose, and a host of other qualities that predict well-being. The Positivity Self Test, another succinct evaluation tool to help clients evaluate their well-being, can be found at *www.PositivityRatio.com*. Barbara Fredrickson (2009) summarizes findings on happiness. She acknowledges that negativity is part of every life and that often clients do not have control over experiences that cause them pain. However, the positive psychology literature suggests that *how* clients respond to life events predicts their overall happiness. For example, Emmons and McCullough (2004) showed that people who kept a daily gratitude journal—writing down what they are grateful for—had high levels of emotional and physical well-being. Other qualities that predict happiness include the capacity to forgive, the ability to achieve "flow" (the ability to immerse oneself in an experience where action and awareness are merged), a balance of daily pleasure and meaning/purpose in life, and the ability to focus on the process of seeking a goal, not just the outcome of achieving a goal such as winning an award or making a large sum of money (Csikszentmihalyi, 1998; Ben-Shahar, 2007). Emotions such as empathy, awe, hope, joy, and pride are associated with a sense of well-being.

Three books that summarize the positivity research and provide assessment tools are *Happier* by Tal Ben-Shahar (2007), which is based on a course he teaches at Harvard about happiness; *Happiness: Unlocking the Mysteries of Psychological Wealth* by Ed Diener and Robert Biswas-Diener (2008), an enjoyable summary of the happiness research that answers questions such as "Can making a lot of money make me happy?" and discusses the important influence of spirituality in finding meaning in life; and *Positivity* by Barbara Fredrickson (2009), which is augmented by the *www.PositivityRatio.com* website.

Both Ben-Shahar (2007) and Fredrickson (2009) suggest using the Day Reconstruction Method developed by Daniel Kahneman and Krueger (2004) to assess client well-being. For this process, clients are asked to:

- Record when you woke up the previous day and when you went to bed.
- Recall your day and divide it into a series of experiences (e.g., got ready for work, met with boss, went for a run). Write down your experiences in order, including how much time they took.

- Review each experience and recall the emotions that you felt during the experience. Write down your feelings as if you are keeping a diary.
- Tally the positive and negative experiences.
- Identify which experiences you'd like to spend more time on and which experiences you'd like to limit.

Meaning, Faith, and Spirituality

Often, clients seek your help as they face deep suffering. It may feel, at times, that you can only offer support to your clients who have pain resulting from traumatic events or devastating losses and empathize as they sometimes draw on deep spiritual reserves of hope and purpose in spite of their pain. Other times, clients seek ways to lead more meaningful, productive lives. Research suggests that faith, spirituality, and religious experience offer sources of solace, meaning, and direction for coping with life's challenges (Diener & Biswas-Diener, 2008; Myers, 2008). In fact, research suggests that religious experience is tied to healthy behaviors such as less smoking and drinking, social support, including strong community ties, and positive emotions including hope and optimism. Thus, part of a comprehensive assessment can be a client's spiritual beliefs and practices. Simply asking about spiritual practice can open up a potential source of well-being that the client may not have initially considered as part of a therapeutic conversation.

Social Isolation versus Social Support

Social isolation and loneliness are additional risk factors. Perhaps the core quality of being human is the need for connection with other human beings. For the last 42 years, George Vaillant has followed 268 men who graduated from Harvard and are now in their eighties or dead. He has sought to understand these men's successes and failures and the measure of their lives. He observed how these men faced life's exigencies.

"It is social aptitude," he writes, "not intellectual brilliance or parental social class that leads to successful aging." Warm connections are necessary—and if not found in a mother or father, they can come from siblings, uncles, friends, mentors. The men's relationships at age 47, he found, predicted later life adjustment better than any other variable except defenses. Good sibling relationships seem especially powerful. Vaillant was asked, "What have you learned from the Grant Study men?" Vaillant's response: "That the only thing that really matters in life are your relationships to other people" (Shenk, 2009, p. 3).

Strong social and emotional ties mean that clients have resources from others when they face challenging times. Attachments buffer clients as they face adversity and in general the personality trait of extraversion is associated with positive mental and physical health outcomes (Cohen, 2004). In fact, increasing social ties creates positive health outcomes such as increased immunity against illness and a sense of wellbeing. In contrast, social isolation and loneliness predict worsening outcomes in mental and physical health.

When evaluating clients, consider their degree of loneliness and isolation. Ask specific questions such as "Do you have someone you could turn to if you needed help?"; "Considering your entire life, who is your closest friend? How often do you talk to or see him?"; "Who knows you the best of all your acquaintances and family members in town? When was the last time you had contact with this person?" "For this specific problem, who has helped you thus far? Who have you talked to about this problem?"

Marriage and Intimate Relationships

David Myers (2000) used research data on well-being to document that there are few stronger predictors of happiness than close, nurturing, equitable, intimate, enduring companionship with one's partner. Sheldon Cohen (2004) summarizes the literature on social support by showing the overwhelming evidence that married people live longer and are healthier. Marriage is a protective factor for men regardless of marital satisfaction. For women, the quality of the marriage, especially equality in decision making and strong companionship, correlates with well-being and positive health (Cohen, 2004; Kiecolt-Glaser & Newton, 2001).

Marriage and family therapists can feel confident that when they assess and treat relationships, they are simultaneously assessing and treating the individuals sitting in their office. Of course, individual assessment of social ties can include work relationships, community ties, spiritual relationships, and others. But, the research is clear that family ties and love account for much of your individual client's well being.

Case Example of Karen, Continued

During her third therapy session, Karen seemed to trust her therapist more. For the first time, Karen talked about her disappointment, anger, and loneliness. Karen felt that her husband had exploited her emotionally throughout their marriage and had exploited her financially during the legal proceedings of the divorce. She said, "Every morning, I wake up and think about how he ruined my life." In addition, Karen reported feeling ashamed that she resented the demands and needs of her daughters and parents. "I know it is my responsibility to help them, but personally, I have no life. I am only a caretaker." Karen had little time for friendship and felt that she would never have a lover again.

As the therapist listened, she made her own list of topics she wanted to eventually discuss with Karen. The therapist's list included:

- Anger/rage at ex-husband
- Boundaries with parents and daughters
- Potential for friendships and dating in the future

The therapist knew that addressing these issues would take time and she wanted to build her relationship with Karen first.

CONCLUSION

This chapter provides guidance on assessment that will help you focus on clients' well-being and daily events, not just assess for psychopathology. Many clients come to therapy because of changes in their lives that cause stress. Other clients seek happier, more fulfilling lives. Most clients seek some information and education about how to have meaningful lives. In conducting assessments of your clients, we hope that you will consider the client's individual goals and needs while simultaneously noting the critical role of fulfilling relationships and love in your clients' lives and in your own life.

CHAPTER 6

Assessing Adults
for Psychopathology

INDIVIDUAL DIAGNOSIS AND THE DSM

Often couples or families will come to therapy with a relationship problem they hope you will help them solve. They describe the problem in terms of changes they want to make in the relationship or changes they want the other person to make. As you carefully listen to their concerns, you also want to consider individual diagnosis. Perhaps one or more family members meet the diagnostic criteria for a specific mental health problem or a "mental health syndrome." One of us was recently involved in a case that demonstrates the interplay between individual and relational diagnosis. Charlotte tells her therapist that she is seriously thinking of divorcing Reese. Her primary complaint is that Reese seldom follows through on the things that he says he will do, which has completely undermined her trust in him. However, as the therapist begins to assess the couple, she soon recognizes that Reese has undiagnosed ADHD, which contributes to his inability to successfully complete many tasks. Addressing his ADHD becomes an important piece of the puzzle in rebuilding the couple's relationship.

According to the DSM, syndromes comprise signs and symptoms. Signs are what you observe in the client. For example, you note that the individual seems agitated or lethargic. Symptoms are concerns that the client reports. For example, the client says that he cannot sleep or that she has no energy. Together, signs and symptoms often cluster together to create syndromes. According to the DSM, syndromes must cause distress or disability or cause an important loss of freedom. In other words, mental health syndromes impede the client's life and cause suffering.

Many therapists do not like to use the DSM for assessment. They believe that no human being can be reduced to a list of signs and symptoms. In addition, the DSM attempts to describe symptoms but doesn't hypothesize about the origins of a problem. Therapists who believe understanding the origins of a problem is essential for effective treatment will be less interested in current signs and symptoms. In addition, many therapists find DSM diagnosis reductionistic. They seek a more comprehensive picture of the client's life that includes understanding more about the client's relationships. While many of these criticisms are warranted, the weaknesses of the DSM are also its strengths.

The DSM can be a concise, albeit reductionistic, guide to important symptoms that the therapist needs to consider. In essence, knowing the DSM criteria alerts the therapist to the possible importance of a symptom (such as a dramatic change in personality) or its potential insignificance (such as a foot itch). Another option is that an initial symptom could be a first hint of a symptom cluster that could be really important (such as a change in sleep pattern that turned into a major depression). Finally, an atypical symptom (such as disorientation in a child) might prompt the therapist to involve other professionals such as a physician. Thus, every therapist should have comprehensive, individual diagnostic skills along with relational assessment skills. The process of determining a specific diagnosis for a client is called differential diagnosis. If you know general categories of disorders, such as mood or anxiety, then you can go a step further and ask, which specific mood disorder does this client have? In addition, you can use the decision trees in Appendix A of the current edition of the DSM—DSM-IV-TR (American Psychiatric Association, 2000)—to help you further refine your diagnosis.

There are many ways to assess for individual psychopathology, including criteria from written checklists or mnemonics, structured interviews, individual and family histories, or client self-report interviews, using a mnemonic, or just listening carefully as the client describes his or her concerns and then asking specific questions related to your hunches about a possible diagnosis. Of these options, the last one offers the best chance of establishing a close therapeutic relationship because it allows a client to tell his or her story. But, this option requires that you have memorized criteria for many individual diagnoses. We recommend you use a combination of these methods. For example, many easily obtained self-report instruments can help ensure the therapist doesn't miss an important diagnosis. In addition, some clients feel reassured about the validity of their diagnoses when they see the results of a "scientific" instrument and they know the assessment follows evidence-based procedures.

Another issue that frequently arises in individual diagnosis is comorbidity (Frances & First, 1995). At times, clients meet criteria for more than one diagnosis. For example, the client might meet criteria for both depression and anxiety. Also, some clients have both a mental health and a physical health problem that are related. For example, clients with irritable bowel syndrome often have clinical depression or anxiety. The therapist wants to identify and document all the possible diagnoses. If possible, he or she also wants to understand the relationships among the different diagnoses. For example:

> Did condition *A* cause condition *B*?
> Did condition *B* cause condition *A*?
> Do *A* and *B* share similar symptoms?
> Is there an underlying condition *C* that causes both *A* and *B*?
> Are *A* and *B* unrelated but co-occurring?

These are some of the key questions you want to consider when making a diagnosis, and one way to do this is to ask questions of time. Which condition came first? When did they start and what else was happening at that time? For example, starting a new medication, either prescribed or illegal, can often result in new conditions or symptoms. One can also consider whether *A* and *B* occur only at the same time, or if they occur separately.

FREQUENCY AND DEMOGRAPHICS OF MENTAL DISORDERS

Knowing the most common diagnoses can be helpful because the therapist knows what to watch for. Also, the therapist knows when clients describe uncommon symptoms. Kessler and his colleagues (Kessler, Berglund, Demler, Jin, & Walters, 2005; Kessler, Chiu, Demler, & Walters, 2005) studied the frequency of different mental disorders in the general population. They gathered data both in the 1990s and the early

2000s. Here are some of the most important findings from these fascinating studies:

- Approximately half of the U.S. population will have a mental disorder at some time in their lives. In the previous 12 months, approximately 30% had a mental disorder.

- A certain group of the population has recurring disorders, often with comorbidity of three or even more disorders. In general, women with little education who are socially isolated and in their 20s or 30s are overrepresented in this group.

- Many disorders start in childhood, especially anxiety problems and behavior disorders such as ADHD. The authors recommend more attention to treating children and adolescents and hope that early intervention can prevent the disorders from becoming lifelong burdens.

- Most people with mental disorders never seek professional treatment, and if they do, they have suffered for several years before they seek professional help. (They may seek to solve their problems in other ways such as talking to friends and family, talking to other professionals such as teachers or religious leaders. Often, if they seek professional help, they go see their primary care doctor, not a therapist.)

- The most common disorders are mood disorders, anxiety disorders, impulse disorders such as ADHD, and substance abuse.

- Women generally have *internalizing disorders* such as depression, in which they turn their feelings in on themselves, while men have *externalizing disorders* and act out in their environment, in ways such as destroying property.

- Predictors for never seeking treatment include being elderly, early age at onset, male, married, low education, minorities, no insurance, and social isolation.

- Marital disruption is associated with many mental health problems.

DIAGNOSTIC GUIDELINES

Over time, expert diagnosticians have identified several principles to help guide the process. For example, therapists should use the most parsimonious diagnosis possible—choose the simplest but most comprehensive diagnosis possible. "Keep it simple" should be your motto when it comes to diagnosis. In addition, therapists should consider issues of safety (Morrison, 2007), such as those discussed in Chapter 4. The six rule-out rules that follow help you systematically evaluate safety issues (Frances & First, 1995). Also, therapists should consider the most common diagnoses described in the previous section before they consider obscure diagnoses. We recommend that you memorize these principles and use them every time you meet a new client. By applying these principles and going through the following steps in a systematic way, therapists can prevent a host of common mistakes.

Rule-Out Rules

The six steps to rule out possible causes of disorders include:

1. *Rule out substance abuse, medications, or toxin exposures.* Failing to consider substances as a cause of mental health symptoms is the most common mistake that therapists make. If the substance is illegal, the client may be reluctant to report using it. If it is a prescribed or legal substance, neither the client nor the therapist may consider it a source of the problem. The client won't know to report using the substance, and the therapist won't consider asking. In addition, toxins like lead, gases, or smoke may be a part of everyday life for the client and thus not a focus of attention. At times, clients might lie about their illegal substance use. If you suspect that your client is lying, ask again later, perhaps waiting until you've built stronger rapport. Questions of time (what happened about the same time as the first symptoms) can often illuminate substance-induced syndromes. Simply ask, "When symptom *x* appeared, had you started taking any new medicines or having any other new experiences in your life?"

2. *Rule out general medical conditions or physical sources for the complaints.* Of course, you are not a physician so you won't be able to completely answer this question. However, you can refer your client to a physician and contact the physician to share your specific questions and concerns. Also, by having a client's health history, you can often discover physical explanations for psychological symptoms. For both substance use and physical illness, therapists often have specific questions asking for this information on their intake forms. For example,

the intake form might ask, "When was your last visit to a physician? What problem did you see the doctor for?" "What medications (prescribed or over-the-counter) are you currently taking?"

3. *Rule out mood disorders.* Mood disorders occur so often that you should still consider them as a possible diagnosis even if a client has dramatic symptoms or meets criteria for another diagnosis. Sometimes, this is difficult because clients with mood disorders present with varied complaints. An elderly man may complain of not enjoying his golf game. An adolescent girl may dramatically change her eating habits. A child may be highly irritable and lose his temper often. The source for all of these changes might be depression. Another reason you want to always consider mood disorders is that depression can lead to suicide. Thus, since one of your primary goals is to keep your clients safe, you want to make sure that you consider a mood disorder as a diagnosis.

4. *Rule out factitious disorder/malingering.* This is another way of saying that you should consider the possibility that your client is faking his or her symptoms. Symptoms may be feigned for a multitude of reasons. As parents, we've dealt with our children's "headaches" when they don't want to go to school and take a test. Sometimes clients cannot face a struggle, dilemma, or trauma in their lives. They may consciously or unconsciously create symptoms to avoid the struggle. Additionally, they may obtain some concrete results—like missing school or some "softer" results like empathy from a partner or parent. At times, the situation becomes more dangerous. For example, Munchausen syndrome by proxy occurs when a parent intentionally makes a child ill in order to receive attention from medical professionals. To avoid missing these complicated, challenging clinical situations, first simply consider the possibility that the client is feigning symptoms.

5. *Do a differential diagnosis.* Once you have a general idea about a possible diagnostic category, for example, anxiety disorders, you should try to distinguish exactly which disorder your client has. In fact, your client may have several anxiety disorders or symptoms from several disorders. As mentioned earlier, Appendix A of DSM-IV-TR can help you with this process. One way to do a differential diagnosis is to list all the possible diagnoses that you want to consider as you listen to clients describe their concerns. Then you can go back and systematically consider each one.

6. *Consider the possibility that your client may not have a specific*

DSM diagnosis. Many other options exist and the client may still need treatment. For example, many children do not meet specific DSM criteria, but they might still need an intervention of some type. Other clients might have some symptoms of a syndrome but not enough for the full diagnosis. In this case, you can't be sure if your client will eventually develop the full syndrome. Other clients may simply be responding to a stressful situation and need support and coping skills. Sometimes clients describe symptoms that are clinically significant but don't fit neatly into a DSM syndrome. Regardless whether your client's symptoms precisely match DSM descriptors, you will want to consider whether your client needs treatment or some type of intervention. If you are not sure, you should consult with your supervisor, get more information, refer your client to an expert, or search the clinical literature for helpful information. One of the most important lessons from this process is that you don't want to become rigid about either diagnosis or treatment protocols.

Below are some clinical scenarios that might have been avoided if the therapists had systematically used the six rule-out rules.

• The therapist told the mother of the adolescent boy that he probably had a psychotic disorder because he had hallucinated. However, the teenager was using illegal drugs, which had caused his symptoms. The therapist failed to consider substance abuse.

• The therapist told the elderly man that he was clinically depressed. His depression made sense because he had recently had a serious cardiovascular illness. The therapist hypothesized that the depression resulted from the client's confrontation with his own mortality. Instead, the man's physician stopped one of the newer medicines he had prescribed for heart disease, and his patient's depression lifted immediately. The therapist had failed to consider the effects of prescribed medications.

• The artist told the therapist that he was having an existential crisis. At times, he felt like he was having an "out-of-body" experience, and he would ponder philosophical issues so intensely that he developed serious headaches. The therapist enjoyed having such a deep, thoughtful client and enjoyed the sessions for 3 months, while the artist's headaches worsened. Eventually, the man was diagnosed with a brain tumor. The therapist failed to consider physical causes for the client's symptoms.

- The therapist told the young woman that she suffered from clinical depression. It made sense that she would be depressed because her marriage was in shambles after she had had two extramarital affairs and secretly maxed out several credit cards. When her husband found out about her deceptions, he raged, her depression worsened, and they decided to start marital therapy. In fact, the woman had a history of reckless behavior, and a psychiatrist diagnosed her with bipolar II. After 2 months on the appropriate medication, her symptoms subsided and her marriage spontaneously improved. The therapist failed to distinguish between different mood disorders to determine the accurate diagnosis.

Mental Status Exam

In addition to the six rule-out rules, other key diagnostic tools exist. One of the most helpful tools is the mental status exam (MSE). The MSE is most commonly used by physicians to understand clients' deficits and their current status. A series of questions evaluates the following areas: judgment, orientation, intellectual functioning, memory, affect (mood), and thought processing. A helpful mnemonic to use when thinking about a client's mental status would be the first letters of the areas that are evaluated—JOIMAT. Formal MSE scores are scored numerically and the client is given an MSE range of mild, moderate, or severe.

The MSE does not indicate why a client has cognitive weaknesses and you may have no idea about etiology. An individual may have dementia, brain trauma, substance abuse effects, a serious medical condition, or a host of other problems that could cause a low MSE score. Most therapists do not have the skills or knowledge to assess etiology. Instead, a therapist would refer the client to a physician with whom he would share his observations and concerns about their mutual client. A therapist may also obtain a history of his client's current symptoms or complaints, including what solutions the client has already tried to ameliorate the problem. In addition, the therapist can get a more detailed history of the client's overall health and life. While the MSE gives a picture of the client's immediate functioning, a history provides a more comprehensive picture.

Many examples of MSEs can be found on the Internet simply by using a search engine. Shortened forms are also available because a full MSE can take 20–30 minutes to administer. While you may not do a full mental status exam often, familiarity with MSEs can help you remember to ask evaluative questions if you suspect a cognitive problem. Simple questions like asking the client what year it is or a simple memory test like asking the client to remember three words (*apple, bicycle, table*) and then asking him or her to repeat the three words 10 minutes later are useful assessment tools to use when you have concerns about the clarity of your client's thinking.

Sometimes clients feel impatient when their doctor "keeps asking me irrelevant questions." In fact, we remember a time when an elderly woman asked her therapist to find her a new doctor. The therapist knew that the physician had an excellent reputation and had seen the caring and concern the doctor demonstrated in his work. The therapist carefully inquired about her client's dissatisfactions. Almost in a whisper, the woman reported that she was suspicious about the doctor's intelligence because he kept asking her what day it was, what city they were in, and who was president—all common questions used to assess orientation in the MSE!

Usually your clients have specific concerns they want to discuss. If you are going to conduct an MSE, you may want to introduce it first by asking permission. For example, you may say, "I want to hear more about your frustrations and disappointments at work. But, first, could I ask you a few questions? They may not seem relevant, but these questions will help me do a better job understanding what you need and how I might help in this situation."

Axes I–V

The editors of the current edition of the DSM (DSM-IV-TR) have responded to critics of the manual who suggest that it is reductionistic by creating a more comprehensive evaluation tool. The multiaxial evaluation system emphasizes biopsychosocial assessment and gives a more comprehensive view of the client. A detailed description of the multiaxal evaluation system can be found in the first few pages of DSM-IV-TR. Here is a brief summary of what is evaluated and recorded on the five sections:

- *Axis I.* Axis I comprises the DSM diagnoses that are the current focus of clinical attention.

- *Axis II: Personality Disorders and Mental Retardation*. One way to think about Axis II compared to Axis I is that in general these disorders are lifelong and more intractable to treatment.

- *Axis III: Clinically Relevant General Medical Conditions*. Physicians have diagnosed these medical problems already and the client reports these conditions to the therapist. It is often important to know about medical conditions because as mentioned earlier, medical illnesses often cause or at least co-occur with mental health symptoms.

- *Axis IV: Psychosocial and Environmental Problems*. In recent years, researchers have clearly documented the damaging effects of stress on clients' mental and physical health. Axis IV is the place to list stressors such as work demands, economic problems, relationship conflicts, and legal struggles. In fact, frequently your clients will want to spend most of their time discussing these stressors, and their motivation for therapy is frequently tied to them.

- *Axis V:* Axis V tries to answer the question "How bad is the problem?" The problem's impact on your client is assessed by considering the following:
  - What is the client's worst symptom (for example, suicide attempts)?
  - How well is the client completing the tasks of daily life (for example, going to work every day)?

In addition, many DSM diagnoses consider length of time the client has been troubled by the syndrome. Evaluating the duration and severity of symptoms and the client's ability to perform normal daily tasks can provide an understanding of the impact of the client's illness and also indicate the urgency of treatment.

COMMONLY USED INSTRUMENTS

Therapists often use screening instruments to quickly identify common syndromes. Many have strong validity and reliability and are easy to score. However, therapists can also misuse screening instruments if they depend on them exclusively to make a diagnosis. Although these instruments can be the first step in a comprehensive diagnostic process, they have the limitations of all self-report instruments. Thus, the therapist's observations, curiosity, questions, and clinical hypotheses should augment the diagnostic process.

It is beyond the scope of this chapter to review all possible instruments that therapists may consider using. Table 6.1 describes popular instruments for some of the most common disorders. Some of these instruments can be downloaded from the Web, while others must be purchased.

SPECIFIC DIAGNOSES INCLUDING MNEMONICS AND SCREENING QUESTIONS

In this section we will review some of the most common DSM diagnoses. As you read about these disorders, remember that you can easily obtain a more detailed description by reading the DSM yourself. In addition, remember that many clients meet criteria for more than one DSM diagnosis, while other clients face significant struggles but have no clear DSM diagnosis. Your assessment should be as comprehensive as possible and not reduced to listening only for DSM symptoms. If you listen carefully to your clients, ask open-ended questions, and, during at least part of the interview, allow them to share their concerns and stories, you are less likely to miss important information. At the same time, knowing the basic criteria for DSM diagnoses will help you identify a specific syndrome when your client starts describing its symptoms.

Many students feel overwhelmed when they first view the DSM. They wonder how they will ever learn the specific criteria for so many disorders. In fact, with each revision of the DSM, more disorders are added. The fourth edition of the DSM describes about three times as many disorders as the first edition described in 1952 (Carey, 2008). Thus, it may be helpful to memorize some mnemonics discussed below for some of the most common disorders and learn some screening questions (Carlat, 1998). The mnemonic phrase "Depressed Patients Seem Anxious So Claim Psychiatrists" is helpful for remembering the major categories of disorders included in the DSM:

- D—Depression including major depression, bipolar disorder, dysthymia
- P—Personality disorders
- S—Substance abuse disorders

TABLE 6.1. Commonly Used Instruments to Screen for Mental Disorders in Adults

Depression

- Beck Depression Inventory II (Beck, Steer, & Brown, 1996)
  www.ibogaine.desk.nl/graphics/3639b1c_23.pdf
- Center for Epidemiologic Studies Depression Scale (CES-D; Radloff, 1977)
  www.chcr.brown.edu/pcoc/cesdscale.pdf
- Cornell Scale for Depression in Dementia (Alexopoulos, Abrams, Young, & Shamoian, 1988)
  qmweb.dads.state.tx.us/Depression/CSDD.htm
- Geriatric Depression Scale (Yesavage et al., 1983)
  www.stanford.edu/~yesavage/GDS.html
- Hamilton Rating Scale for Depression (Hamilton, 1960)
  healthnet.umassmed.edu/mhealth/HAMD.pdf
- PHQ2 and PHQ9 (Spitzer, Kroenke, & Williams, 1999)
  www.docsfortots.org/documents/phqscreeningtool.pdf (PHQ2)
  www.americangeriatrics.org/education/dep_tool_05.pdf (PHQ9)
- Zung Self-Rating Depression Scale (Zung, 1965)
  healthnet.umassmed.edu/mhealth/ZungSelfRatedDepressionScale.pdf

Anxiety

- Beck Anxiety Inventory (Beck, Epstein, Brown, & Steer, 1988).
  www.myonlinetherapy.com/Therapists/Documents/Beck%20Anxiety%20Inventory.doc
- Duke Anxiety–Depression Scale (DUKE-AD; Parkerson & Broadhead, 1997)
  http://healthmeasures.mc.duke.edu/images/DukeAD.pdf
- Hamilton Anxiety Scale (HAMA; Hamilton, 1959)
  http://www.sommeil-mg.net/spip/questionnaires/HAM_A.pdf
- Social Phobia Inventory (SPIN; Connor et al., 2000)
  http://www.drjenna.net/checklists/anxiety/social_phobia_inventory.pdf

Diagnostic interviews for adults

- Structured Clinical Interview for DSM Disorders (SCID; Spitzer, Williams, Gibbon, & First, 1992)
  cpmcnet.columbia.edu/dept/scid/faq/scid_2.html

General psychiatric assessment measures

- Brief Symptom Inventory (BSI; Derogatis, 1993)
  psychcorp.pearsonassessments.com/HAIWEB/Cultures/en-us/Productdetail.htm?Pid=PAbsi&Mode=summary
- Mental Health Inventory (MHI; Veit & Ware, 1983)
  www.rand.org/health/surveys_tools/mos/mos_mentalhealth_survey.pdf
- PRIME-MD–PHQ (Spitzer, Williams, Kroenke, Linzer, & Verloin deGruy, 1994)
  www.montana.edu/wwwebm/Archives/PHQ.doc
- SCL-90-R (Lucht, Jahn, Barnow, & Freyberger, 2002).
  www.pearsonassessments.com/scl90.aspx

(continued)

TABLE 6.1. (*continued*)

Substance abuse

- CAGE (Ewing, 1984)
  www.ssdha.nshealth.ca/SSH%20CAGE%20_2_.pdf
- Michigan Alcoholism Screening Test (MAST; Selzer, 1971)
  www.ncadd-sfv.org/downloads/mast_test.pdf
- TWEAK (Russell, 1994)
  pubs.niaaa.nih.gov/publications/Assesing%20Alcohol/InstrumentPDFs/74_TWEAK.pdf

Note. Websites provide examples of the instruments or the publisher's home page.

- <u>A</u>—Anxiety disorders including panic with agoraphobia, obsessive–compulsive disorder
- <u>S</u>—Somatization disorder/eating disorders—both involve disorders of bodily perception
- <u>C</u>—Cognitive disorders including dementia, delirium
- <u>P</u>—Psychotic disorders including schizophrenia, delusional disorder, and psychosis accompanying depression, substance abuse, or dementia

When you use mnemonics, remember to simultaneously keep building rapport with your client. For example, you can normalize clients' behaviors and demonstrate empathy for their plight. Also, you can ask the questions in a way that gently assumes the client may already demonstrate the symptom. Finally, you can try to keep the assessment conversational in tone instead of abruptly moving from topic to topic.

Mood Disorders

For clients, mood struggles frequently co-occur with other problems they might have. Also, mood disorders frequently accompany physical health problems. For example, coronary heart disease, cancer, and immune-function disorders are often comorbid with depression. An initial screening question you can ask your clients if you suspect a mood disorder is: "Are you depressed and sad?" Depression refers to a lasting feeling of hopelessness, sadness, and loss of pleasure and energy. SIGE-CAPS (what a doctor's prescription may look like: SIG: Energy CAP-Sules) is a useful mnemonic for remembering the eight neurovegetative symptoms of depression:

- S—Sleep disorder (either increased or decreased sleep)
- I—Interest deficit (anhedonia)
- G—Guilt (worthlessness, hopelessness, regret)
- E—Energy deficit
- C—Concentration deficit
- A—Appetite disorder (either increased or decreased appetite)
- P—Psychomotor retardation or agitation
- S—Suicidality

When you have depressed clients, always consider the possibility that they may want to kill themselves. We describe demographic predictors of suicide and skills for evaluating suicide risk in Chapter 4. In addition, "IS PATH WARM?" can be a helpful mnemonic for assessing suicide risk factors:

- I—Ideation
- S—Substance abuse
- P—Purposelessness
- A—Anxiety
- T—Trapped
- H—Hopelessness
- W—Withdrawal
- A—Anger
- R—Recklessness
- M—Mood change

Mood disorders may also include mania. Mania describes a period of persistently elevated, expansive, or irritable mood. The mnemonic DIGFAST describes the key symptoms of mania:

- D—Distractibility
- I—Indiscretion (excessive involvement in pleasurable activities)
- G—Grandiosity
- F—Flight of ideas
- A—Activity increase
- S—Sleep (decreased need for sleep)
- T—Talkativeness (pressured-speech)

In order to screen for manic episodes when assessing a client who may have bipolar disorder, you can ask: "Have you had periods of feeling so happy or energetic that your friends said you were talking too fast or that you were too 'hyper'?" Clients who have experienced both periods of depressed mood and periods of mania are diagnosed with bipolar disorder. At times clients may alternate between both mood extremes or even show symptoms of both in the same day (mixed episodes). In addition, some clients have mild depression or mild manic symptoms (hypomania), and each of these variations guides the process of differential diagnosis.

Mood disorders can remain unrecognized and untreated for years and can cause deep suffering for clients and their loved ones. Families struggle with how to help their depressed member and at times resent the effects of the client's depression on their lives. Both depression and mania are treatable. While research suggests that bipolar disorder is seldom "cured," both depressed and manic clients can obtain effective treatments that ameliorate their suffering and prevent suicide. Identifying depressed or manic clients and helping them obtain evidence-based treatments can change the course of their lives.

Anxiety (Fears and Worries)

Underlying anxiety disorders is a sense of fear and worry (Anxiety Disorders Association of America, 2009). Many anxiety disorders are characterized by feelings of helplessness and loss of control. Physical complaints such as rapid heartbeat, sweating, trembling, or breathlessness lead many anxious individuals to seek help from a physician, not a therapist. Family therapists should pay special attention to anxiety disorders because anxiety seems to run in families. Whether the etiology is biological (genetic) or learned, when one family member has an anxiety disorder, others often have symptoms. If you evaluate a child for an anxiety disorder, you should also consider evaluating his or her parents. Anxiety disorders usually start at a young age, around eleven years old, and children seldom receives any treatment for them. Thus, by the time they are adults, fear and worry have become a way of life and they are even less likely to seek treatment.

Several specific disorders are included under the broad category of anxiety in the DSM. Refer to the DSM to learn more about generalized anxiety disorder, panic disorder (with or without agoraphobia), obsessive–compulsive disorder, posttraumatic stress disorder, and phobias, including social phobia. The following are useful screening questions for several of the disorders:

Obsessive–compulsive disorder

"Do you have thoughts that bother you or make you anxious that
   you can't get rid of regardless of how hard you try?"
"Do you have a tendency to keep things extremely clean and to wash
   your hands more frequently than other people you know?"
"Do you check things over and over to excess?"

Posttraumatic Stress disorder

"Have you experienced or witnessed a life-threatening event that
   caused intense fear, helplessness, or horror?"
"Do you reexperience the event?"

Panic disorder

"Are you troubled by repeated, unexpected 'attacks' during which
   you suddenly are overcome by intense fear or discomfort for no
   apparent reason?"
"During these attacks, do you experience symptoms such as pound-
   ing heart, sweating, trembling, shortness of breath, or choking
   or other physical symptoms?"

Social phobia

"Does fear of embarrassment cause you to avoid doing things or
   speaking to people?"
"Do you avoid activities in which you are the center of attention?"
"Is being embarrassed or looking stupid among your worst fears?"

In addition, key general screening questions can help you initially
identify specific disorders (for example: "Do you tend to be an anxious
or nervous person?"). Also, many brief self-report and interview instruments are available that screen for specific anxiety disorders. Table 6.1
lists some of the best anxiety screening instruments.

While the DSM separates symptoms of anxiety into specific diagnoses, your clients will probably have symptoms from several disorders.
For example, your client may have panic attacks and some obsessions
but not meet the full criteria for either panic disorder or obsessive–
compulsive disorder. Also, anxious clients' primary symptoms and chief
complaints often vary over time. Anxious clients are often depressed,
and they may abuse substances to treat their anxiety. For example, a

college student with social phobia may regularly get drunk before he can go to a party.

Regardless of the client's specific anxiety disorder, he or she usually shares a common response with other anxious clients—avoidance. A client may avoid touching doorknobs and compulsively wash his hands. Another client may refuse to leave her house. A lonely, anxious individual may give excuses to avoid going to parties, even when he longs for social contact. A client who was raped may avoid all interaction with men. Regardless of the disorder, anxious individuals avoid situations where they feel threatened and in general avoid any situation where they perceive risk. When questioned, the clients may realize that their fears are unwarranted but they may still be unable to face these fears. These same clients may furtively hide their "strange" behaviors because they recognize that their behaviors and fears are extreme.

Cognitive (Thinking and Memory)

The section in the DSM on cognitive disorders used to be called organic disorders because these disorders were thought to have a biological etiology and other disorders were considered "functional." Now, the editors of the DSM recognize that distinguishing between biological and functional etiology is a false dichotomy. Instead, all disorders are viewed through the lens of the biopsychosocial model. Nevertheless, cognitive disorders including dementia, delirium, and amnestic disorder have strong biological underpinnings.

Cognitive disorders involve losses in memory and executive functioning, or thinking skills. The ability to organize, plan, sequence, recall the past, consider the future, and juggle daily responsibilities and other brain functions are lost. Often, these clients are confused, and their families are confused about the changes occurring in their loved one. Often the ability to learn new facts and create new memories is impaired. Short-term memories are no longer formed and older memories begin to dissipate. Depending on the etiology of the cognitive decline, the changes may be temporary or permanent. Specific skills and knowledge are lost, while other areas of the brain remain unchanged. While delirium can often be treated and corrected, a diagnosis of dementia usually implies a gradual, irreversible decline eventually resulting in death.

Therapists can use the MSE to screen for cognitive disorders or use only parts of it. For example, a therapist may ask, "Where are we right now?"; " What day is today?" Another option, mentioned earlier when describing the MSE, is for the therapist to repeat three words—*ball, chair, purple*—and ask the client to memorize these words for later recall. Then the therapist can ask the client to repeat the three memorized words after 10 minutes have passed. A final option is to ask the client to draw a clock face with the time: ten minutes after ten. Clients with cognitive deficits often have trouble completing this task.

Cognitive disorders that involve permanent biological changes, such as plaques and tangles in the brain, may seem like the purview of physicians. Indeed, for these disorders in particular, therapists should collaborate with physicians, who may provide the initial diagnosis. Delirium, in particular, is often a medical emergency, and delirious clients need a medical assessment quickly. However, once the diagnosis is made, cure is often not a possibility for many cognitive disorders. Instead, family therapists can conduct a new assessment of the client's and family's extant resources. Both clients and their caregivers face many challenges as they plan for the future and seek to balance the needs of their vulnerable family member with the needs of the rest of the family.

Adult ADHD

While it is beyond the scope of this chapter to consider all the diagnoses listed under impulse disorders, adult ADHD warrants noting because it is common in adulthood but frequently missed by clinicians (Kessler et. al., 2006). Chapter 8 provides more detail on ADHD in childhood. ADHD continues into adulthood for many clients. Often, the most apparent symptom, hyperactivity, dissipates, while inattention and impulsivity continue. Thus, adults with ADHD often have disrupted relationships, vocational instability, poor driving records, and legal struggles. If a client wasn't diagnosed with ADHD in childhood, he may start therapy because of his struggles. For example, he may complain about career problems, or his family members may complain about his interpersonal difficulties.

Some key screening questions developed by the World Health Organization for Adult ADHD include:

> "How often do you have trouble wrapping up the final details of a project once the challenging parts have been done?"

"How often do you have difficulty getting things in order when you have to do a task that requires organization?"

"How often do you have problems remembering appointments or obligations?"

"When you have a task that requires a lot of thought, how often do you avoid or delay getting started?"

"How often do you fidget or squirm with your hands or feet when you have to sit down for a long time?"

"How often do you feel overly active and compelled to do things, like you were driven by a motor?" (Kessler et al., 2005).

These questions are scored using a range of responses: never, rarely, sometimes, often, and very often. If your client responds affirmatively to several of these questions, consider a referral to an expert in ADHD.

Substance Use (Abuse and Dependence)

Substance abuse is often hidden. Clients seldom initially complain about their substance abuse and may lie to hide it even when the therapist asks directly. In addition, clients will minimize their use or deny that the substance use should be the focus of clinical attention. Thus, William Miller and his colleagues have developed *motivational interviewing*—an assessment style that helps the therapist join with the client's concerns instead of getting in a power struggle about the goals of therapy (Miller & Rollnick, 2002). Using motivational interviewing, a therapist evaluates if the client has a substance use problem, but equally important, the therapist evaluates if the client wants to change his or her substance use at this point in time. Both are important components of assessment.

An initial screening question that is useful in assessing for alcohol abuse is: "Do you have a drink now and then?" The CAGE mnemonic (Ewing, 1984) offers four key questions to screen for alcohol use. Answering yes to two or more of the following questions may indicate a substance problem:

"Have you ever felt you ought to Cut down on your drinking?"

"Have people Annoyed you by criticizing your drinking?"

"Have you ever felt bad or Guilty about your drinking?"

"Have you ever had a drink first thing in the morning to steady your nerves or get rid of a hangover (Eye opener)?"

Other instruments to consider include the Michigan Alcohol Screening Test (MAST; Selzer, 1971), and the TWEAK (Russell, 1994). The MAST has been widely used for many years. The TWEAK is targeted toward women and easy to use as a first-step screening instrument. Both instruments are mentioned in Table 6.1.

In addition, many valid instruments for helping the client do his or her own self-assessment can be found on websites like www. rethinkingdrinking.niaa.nih.gov. However, as mentioned earlier, the most common mistake made when it comes to substance assessment is not asking about substance use at all, especially when the client has complaints that initially seem unrelated to substance use. While not always immediately apparent, substance use makes many other disorders worse and complicates the clinical picture.

Substance use can include a pattern of tolerance (needing more of the substance to get the same effect), withdrawal (biological and emotional symptoms from stopping the substance), and compulsive use. Substance abusers often start using larger amounts than they intended, have trouble controlling their use over time, eventually organize their lives and relationships around the substance, and ultimately give up their relationships, jobs, and lives in order to keep using the substance.

Psychosis

Psychotic disorders are less common than many of the other disorders and often easier to spot because of the *positive symptoms*. These symptoms aren't positive in the sense of being desirables. They are positive in that they are added to a person's life and not seen in healthy people. The positive symptoms include delusions (false beliefs), hallucinations (false sensory experiences), disorganized speech, and disorganized behavior. Usually psychotic individuals also have *negative symptoms*, which involve something that has been lost. Common negative symptoms include the loss of purpose or will, the loss of fluent speech, and the loss of a full range of emotions.

A diagnosis of psychosis should be given by an experienced clinician because of its serious implications. Many psychotic disorders, including schizophrenia, cannot be cured, and the troubled clients with these disorders often face a life of incapacity. The illness limits their ability to work, maintain relationships, and lead a productive life. When they are not actively psychotic, clients often recognize these deficits and feel a profound sense of loss. We have had some of our most moving interviews with stable clients with psychoses who long to achieve normal milestones—a simple, stable job, a caring relationship. At other times, such individuals are out of touch with reality, and their psychotic episodes are often medical emergencies where hospitalization, even if temporary, is the only option. Even more painful situations exist when psychotic clients have exhausted family support and government benefits and are homeless.

Like clients with cognitive disorders, psychotic individuals challenge the resources and energy of their family members. In fact, the origins of family therapy included evaluating the characteristics of families with schizophrenic members. Boundaries/overinvolvement and hostility/criticism are two important family qualities that seem to affect schizophrenic family members. David Milkowitz has developed a program to assess and treat individuals with serious mental illness such as schizophrenia and bipolar disorder (Milkowitz, 2008). While family therapists often seek the expertise of physicians for diagnosing psychotic disorders, assessment of the family interaction, which may be equally important, can be done by a family therapist. Research suggests that supportive families with appropriate boundaries can often help psychotic family members. Even though there is strong research support for biological origins to these challenging disorders, psychosocial assessment and treatments affect the course of the illness and the life course of the client.

In addition, it is important for family therapists to keep in mind that some individuals are at increased risk for psychosis. These include clients with a diagnosis of major depression, substance abuse, or dementia and clients who are guarded, suspicious, or otherwise odd. It may be useful for family therapists to use the following screening questions when assessing for psychotic disorders: "Depression sometimes causes people to have strange experiences, like hearing voices or feeling that others are trying to harm them. Has that happened to you?" "When you misplace things, do you sometimes think that they've been stolen?" If the client answers yes, help him or her get an appointment with a psychiatrist for a more complete evaluation.

Personality Disorders

Personality disorders are "a lasting pattern of behavior and inner experience that markedly deviates from norms of the client's culture" (American Psychiatric Association, 2000, p. 685). The mnemonic I DESPAIRR describes the characteristics of one of the most common personality disorders, borderline personality disorder.

- <u>I</u>—Identity problem
- <u>D</u>—Disordered affect
- <u>E</u>—Empty feeling
- <u>S</u>—Suicidal behavior
- <u>P</u>—Paranoia or dissociative symptoms
- <u>A</u>—Abandonment terror
- <u>I</u>—Impulsivity
- <u>R</u>—Rage
- <u>R</u>—Relationship instability

There are currently 10 specific personality disorders in the DSM[1] and they are clustered according to specific themes. Clients with Cluster A personalities appear odd or eccentric (paranoid, schizoid, and schizotypal). Cluster B includes disorders characterized by dramatic, emotional, and erratic behaviors (antisocial, borderline, histrionic, and narcissistic). Cluster C includes dependent, avoidant and obsessive–compulsive personalities, and these clients often appear anxious or fearful.

Often, therapists are busy assessing a client for another disorder such as depression when they notice self-defeating patterns of behavior that the client keeps repeating regardless of the consequences. Other times, the therapist notes that initial attempts at assessment or treatment are not working and building the therapeutic relationship seems fraught with challenges. Thus, personality disorders are often not the focus of initial assessment, but instead, over time, they come into focus as an explanation for complicated clinical situations. The risk in this process is that anytime a therapist is perplexed, he or she may inadvertently jump to assessing the client for a personality disorder instead of looking for alternative explanations.

Many controversies surround both diagnosis and treatment of clients with personality disorders. But, in general, clinicians agree on a few points. First, personality disorders are thought to develop early in life and remain stable over time and across settings. These are lifelong patterns of behavior, thought, and emotion. In addition, these patterns must cause distress and have negative consequences in the client's life.

---

[1] See *www.dsm5.org* for a proposed reformulation of personality disorders in the DSM-5.

Relationships, work, family life, and other areas are negatively affected by the effects of the personality disorder. The presence of a personality disorder in your client will often complicate both the assessment and treatment of the client's primary complaint.

Other Disorders

The brief description above covers some of the most common categories of mental disorders but is not exhaustive. Somatization disorder, dissociative disorders, and impulse control disorders are just a few of the DSM syndromes not discussed above. We recommend that you become familiar with the DSM. Reading a casebook that offers vignettes describing different disorders is an engaging way to learn the sometimes dry descriptors included in the DSM. While your assessments should extend beyond DSM diagnoses, you should be familiar with the categories of the DSM so you can identify mental health problems in your clients and their families while simultaneously assessing them from multiple perspectives.

INDIVIDUAL AND FAMILY DIAGNOSIS

As family therapists, we must be mindful of the interplay between individual diagnoses and couple or family dynamics. An individual's mental illness can negatively impact the quality of couple or family relationships. Conversely, the quality of these relationships can also impact the course of that mental illness. Tyson, 52, and Annabelle, 49, presented in therapy because of conflict and emotional distance in their marriage. Tyson, who had long suffered from bouts of depression, was recently diagnosed with bipolar II disorder. When Tyson had particularly bad days struggling with bipolar symptoms, he would become overly critical of Annabelle. Annabelle responded to his criticism by withdrawing. Tyson felt isolated and lonely when she withdrew, which only made his mood state worse.

We recommend that you stay abreast of the emerging research on the interface between family diagnosis and individual health. Research demonstrates that family interaction and transitions affect physical and mental health for many years after the actual events. For example, divorce and widowhood can have lasting effects on individuals' health, and divorced or widowed people have 20 percent more chronic health conditions such as heart disease, diabetes, and cancer than married people (Waite & Hughes, 2009). Indeed, Christakis and Fowler (2009) have demonstrated that our social ties, particularly our close relationships, can affect our health and well-being in myriad ways. "People are connected, and so their health is connected ... health improvements in one person might spread to others" (Christakis & Fowler, 2007, p. 5). For example, happiness, loneliness, obesity, and smoking are four areas where our relationships strongly influence our behavior.

In recent years, family scholars have tried to tease out the unique influences of family interaction on the development of psychopathology. While a solid body of research demonstrates the power of close family relationships in predicting happiness and well-being, discussions continue on the role of family interaction in the development of psychopathology (Beach, Wamboldt, Kaslow, Heyman, & Reiss, 2006; Myers, 2000). Perhaps one result of these discussions will be the inclusion of relational diagnoses in future revisions of the DSM.

Beach and colleagues (Beach, Wamboldt, Kaslow, Heyman, & Reiss, 2006; Beach, Wamboldt, Kaslow, Heyman, First, et al., 2006) describe relational processes that influence psychopathology. They do not argue for including family patterns such as abusive parenting or serious marital discord as distinct disorders in the DSM. Instead, they recommend that the connections between relational processes and disorders be included. For example, research links marital conflict and ongoing depressive symptoms. In addition conflict between parents and children and weak emotional parent–child bonds influence the development of psychopathology and the capacity to cope with stressful life events. We recommend that you stay abreast of developments in individual diagnosis and simultaneously incorporate emerging research on family diagnosis into your assessment process.

CONCLUSION

For most therapists and clients, clinical diagnosis is only one part of a comprehensive assessment and treatment plan. But, it can be an important part because obtaining an accurate diagnosis can lead to specific evidence-based treatments including psychotropic medications. While your clients need to know that you understand and value their emotions and experiences, we recommend that you simultaneously evaluate them for specific diagnoses.

CHAPTER 7

Assessing Children and Adolescents

In the previous two chapters, we have looked at how to assess adults, including how to evaluate for possible mental disorders. Our attention now turns to assessing children and adolescents. As with assessment of adults, we divide our discussion of children and adolescents into two chapters. This chapter discusses how to assess youth in general, while Chapter 8 examines mental disorders common to children and adolescents.

Although many of the skills used with adults will transfer to the assessment of children and adolescents, there are some critical differences. An additional set of skills and knowledge is necessary to successfully work with this population. Therefore, we begin by exploring how assessment of children and adolescents can be different from working with adults. Next we describe the important areas to assess when evaluating child and adolescent functioning and illustrate this with two case examples, one with a child and one with an adolescent. The chapter concludes with a brief discussion of assessment instruments that can be used to evaluate child and adolescent functioning.

Although this chapter focuses on assessing individual children or adolescents, it is important to stress that we believe child and adolescent assessment needs to be done concurrently with family assessment (see Chapters 9 and 10). All individuals are shaped by the relational context in which they live. This is particularly true for children and adolescents. A failure to include the family dynamics in the assessment of children and adolescents provides an incomplete picture and is a disservice to the youth you are treating.

SPECIAL ISSUES IN ASSESSING CHILDREN AND ADOLESCENTS

Individuals working with youth will need to approach assessment differently than they do with adults. Some of these differences are discussed below.

Play Therapy

Therapists who treat children, particularly young children, may use play therapy in their work. Although play therapy is most often used with young children, it can also be used with adolescents and adults and can be viewed as a form of both assessment and treatment. Play therapy as a form of assessment is addressed here.

A variety of techniques can be used in play therapy. Allowing a child to play with various types of toys (e.g., dollhouses, action figures, kitchen) provides a window into his or her life. Puppets and sand trays are other popular forms of play therapy.

Play therapy has several advantages. First, it can be a fun way for a child to engage in therapy. Second, it has been said that play is the language of children. Particularly for younger children who may have difficulty with verbal expression, play can be a medium for communicating about their inner life. Third, play may be a safe way to explore sensitive topics. For example, by projecting his or her feelings onto a puppet, a child may be able to express something that he or she would have a difficult time owning or saying directly.

When doing play therapy, you must decide whether it will be directive or nondirective. In directive play, the therapist chooses the activity for the child, and may even attempt to guide the child toward addressing certain topics. A therapist who wants to understand a child's perspective on the family may ask the child to play with a dollhouse that includes a family set of dolls or figures. Nondirective play allows the child choose the form of play and is the equivalent of an open-ended question, giving children the freedom to express themselves in any manner they choose.

A key challenge in play therapy is figuring out how to interpret the information that you observe. In some cases, the therapeutic theme or issue may be relatively easy to see. Keysha, a 9-year-old girl, was asked by her therapist to pick out some toys from the shelf for play in the sand tray. Very quickly she grabbed several animals, mostly dinosaurs, and took them to the tray. She also chose a small bridge, which she put in the center of the tray with animals on both sides. She said, "The animals were at war and always fighting." The war seemed to represent the conflict occurring between her parents, who had been separated for the past 3 months. However, in some circumstances, it may be difficult to discern what meaning, if any, should be attributed to the child's play. Is the little boy who has a superhero defeating a bad guy during his play metaphorically expressing his need for protection from someone harming him, or is he simply acting out a cartoon episode that he saw recently?

Given the subjective and difficult nature of interpreting play therapy information, it is important to seek the proper training and education when using this approach. In addition, any themes or hypotheses generated through play therapy should be confirmed through other means (e.g., interviewing parents, observing family dynamics).

Drawings

Drawings can be another important tool in assessing children and to a lesser extent, adolescents. The House–Tree–Person test (Buck, 1977) and Kinetic Family Drawing technique (Burns & Kaufman, 1972) both use drawings clinically, with the help of an interpretative manual. In a Kinetic Family Drawing, the child is asked to draw his or her family doing something. Hypotheses about family dynamics can be derived from this. For example, one can observe which "family members" are included or excluded in the drawing. When asked to do a drawing, Kendra did not include her stepfather or stepsiblings in her drawing even though they were living in the household. One can also observe the child's position and size relative to other family members. Does he or she seem to be an integral part of the family, or does he or she seem marginalized? Is there a sense of unity or closeness in the family? Are they doing a shared activity, or is everyone doing separate activities (perhaps suggesting disengagement in some cases). One should also pay careful attention to what emotions family members seem to be experiencing, especially the child.

As with play therapy, interpretation is subjective and should be done with great caution. Sometimes, however, the meaning of the picture is easy to see. Robert, age 10, was brought into therapy for behavioral issues by his mother, Rebecca. Rebecca had recently married Joseph, who brought with him his son Jacob from a previous marriage. When asked to do a Kinetic Family Drawing, Robert drew his family playing baseball. The "home" team, which consisted of himself and his mother, was beating the "visiting team" (Joseph and Jacob) by a score of 100 to 0. After viewing the drawing, the therapist hypothesized that Robert was struggling with the addition of the new family members, whom he viewed as intruders into his family.

Activities

Including activities in therapy can also facilitate assessment. Obviously play therapy can be one type of activity. However, you may also want to incorporate other activities without the express purpose of having them be play therapy. Children and younger adolescents may be more likely to engage in therapy if it centers on an activity such as a board game. One therapist was having difficulty engaging an adolescent in conversation until they began to play a game of Jenga. This strategy may be particularly helpful for boys, who, like adult males, bond by sharing activities. Boys who are reluctant to talk may open up while playing a game or doing some other activity. You should also be alert to the possible assessment information that comes out in how the client engages in the activity, and not just the conversation that accompanies it. For example, how a child reacts to losing or winning a game may have significance.

Reliance on Other Reporters

Although getting other perspectives is important in working with adults, it is essential in working with children and adolescents. Young children may lack the language and cognitive development to clearly articulate what they are experiencing. They may also have difficulty accurately reporting their behavior. Adolescents may not be completely truthful or forthcoming in sharing information, and need to have their report cross-checked with others. Thus, getting information from adults who are involved in the child's or adolescent's life is necessary to gain a complete and accurate picture.

The obvious adults to include in your assessment are the parents or caregivers. However, other adults may also have an important perspective. Teachers spend a significant amount of time with children and may have important insights about them. Other relatives (e.g., grandparents, aunts, uncles) may also be able to share helpful observations. In some cases, an adolescent's friend or boyfriend/girlfriend may be able to provide helpful information.

Developmental Issues in Assessment

Conducting an effective assessment with children or adolescents requires having a proper knowledge of developmental issues. This is critical for a number of reasons. First, a knowledge of developmental issues will help you tune in to what may be pressing concerns for someone your client's age. A young child will have very different issues and needs from those of an adolescent. Adolescents, for example, may be very concerned about changes in their body as they mature, and with dating or sexuality. Adolescents also have a greater need to develop their own identity, which may lead them to experiment and sometimes resist parental influences.

A sound knowledge of child and adolescent development is also necessary to properly evaluate if your client's behavior is normal or not. Failure to consider your client's developmental stage can lead to one of two possible errors. One is to overpathologize something that is developmentally normal for a child that age. Identifying a 16-year-old talking back to her parents as "oppositional and deviant behavior" might be overstated. It could simply be a part of normal adolescent development that includes the desire to identify one's beliefs and separate them from those of one's parents. The opposite mistake is to overlook a problem because one does not recognize the client is developmentally delayed. One therapist, who had limited experience with young children, did not recognize that Eric, a 3½ year-old boy, was delayed in his speech development. However, his preschool teacher recognized that his speech was delayed and suggested that he be formally evaluated. A formal evaluation confirmed a delay in speech and language, which resulted in Eric getting appropriate services.

Therapists with limited experience working with children may be unsure as to what is developmentally appropriate. In these cases, it is important to seek out supervision from someone who has a solid knowledge of child development. As the above example of Eric suggests, consulting with teachers may also give you clues your client is behind developmentally, since they can compare the child to other children of a similar age.

It may be difficult for you to know how aggressively to treat some issues. Will the child normally outgrow the issue, or does it require intervention so the child's future development is not limited or impacted? This may be a difficult question to answer in some circumstances. Certain young children will naturally outgrow some shyness as they mature, whereas others may need special help or assistance to overcome their shyness. Again, getting supervision or consultation with someone knowledgeable about child development can assist you in making these difficult judgments.

The way in which you conduct assessment will also depend upon the developmental level of your client. Traditional talk therapy is often feasible with older adolescents. However, incorporation of an activity or play therapy is usually necessary for younger clients. Your questions will also need to match the client's developmental level. You cannot ask a young child the same type of questions that you can ask an adult. Young children are concrete thinkers and cannot answer questions that require abstract thinking in the way that adults can.

CHALLENGES IN ASSESSING ADOLESCENTS

Kevin, a 17-year-old senior in high school, was told by his mother that he had to go to counseling, or she would take away his driving privileges. His mother was concerned about his poor school attendance (he occasionally skipped classes or came late to school) and his failure to follow the rules at home, such as staying out late or not doing chores. His mother was also concerned he had seemed moody and irritable ever since his parents had divorced when he was 14. Kevin reluctantly agreed to go to one counseling session.

The therapist is presented with a problem in this case. There is obviously a power struggle between Kevin and his mother. She is giving him an ultimatum with regard to counseling, and he is responding with a willingness to only go once. This struggle can impede the therapist's assessment, since Kevin is coming to therapy with a time limit in his mind.

Joining with Kevin first is the best approach. Initially, it would be important to let him tell his story without being judged or corrected. The therapist would not want to take sides, but rather remain neutral toward Kevin and his mother and try to understand Kevin's perspective. Once he feels somewhat safe and understood, the therapist can attempt to access areas where he is vulnerable. Using probing questions interspersed with empathy will help to make this possible. An example might be "It must have been hard for you when you parents separated. What changed?" This could be followed up with questions about his feelings. If he says that he doesn't know or withdraws, then the therapist might change the topic and suggest, "We can come back to that later." It will be useful for the therapist to be respectful and help the adolescent to maintain a feeling of control in the session. Since Kevin is already in a power struggle with his mother, it is important not to re-create it in the therapy. Ideally, participating in therapy should feel like it is his choice. It might be useful to try and elicit experiences or feelings that he might benefit from talking about. You might ask questions like, "What might you be interested in changing or learning about yourself that could prove useful?"

In addition to the lack of motivation exemplified in Kevin's case, other challenges in assessing adolescents can include a desire to be private, reluctance to talk, or taking a very protective or defensive stance. These areas are best approached on a case-by-case basis, but the process is essentially the same. Joining with adolescents comes first. The therapist needs to develop rapport. Help them to feel comfortable and find a window into their world. Don't assume that you know about them. Let them tell you. Understanding is a key to lowering their reluctance to open up. How quickly this occurs will depend more on their desire to do so than it does on therapeutic techniques. Your task is to assess the level of difficulties the adolescent is experiencing and to evaluate the impact they are having on the client's functioning. It will then be possible to determine if therapy would be useful and what mode of working is likely to be most effective.

ASSESSING CHILD
AND ADOLESCENT FUNCTIONING

Embry, a 16-year-old male, tells you in the first session that he is fine and does not need therapy. You learn that he is mandated to come to therapy because he was caught with a small amount of marijuana after leaving a party. He denies having a drug problem and states he uses marijuana only recreationally and does not abuse drugs like other kids he knows. Do you agree with Embry that he is fine and does not need therapy? What will help you answer this question?

Aside from further investigating Embry's drug use, you will need to consider how well Embry is doing in other areas of his life. Is his marijuana use impacting him in any way, such as in school? Or, is he using marijuana as a way to cope with problems in other areas of his life?

You must be able to effectively assess Embry in multiple areas to conduct a proper assessment. Remembering that children and adolescents are JUST PEOPLE will help you in your assessment. JUST PEOPLE (see Table 7.1) is a mnemonic that we have developed to help us recall the key areas we need to examine to be thorough in our assessment. Evaluating functioning in each of these areas can uncover both strengths and areas of concern. Depending upon the nature of the case, you may discover that some areas are highly salient, while others are of minimal importance.

Although JUST PEOPLE outlines areas for assessing child and adolescent functioning, most of these areas could also apply to adults, especially young adults. (Occupational functioning rather than education would likely be the more salient concern for adults.) Therefore, JUST PEOPLE could be used with adults, but its application would be somewhat different from the way it is used for children and adolescents, since they are at different developmental stages. So, the questions that one might ask within each area can depend upon whether the client is a child, adolescent, or adult.

TABLE 7.1. Checklist for Evaluating Child and Adolescent Functioning Using JUST PEOPLE

- Judgment
- Understanding of others
- Self-esteem
- Temperament
- Peers
- Emotions
- Outside interests
- Psychopathology
- Loved ones
- Education

Judgment

Does your client show good judgment? For example, does your client seem immature or appropriately mature for his or her age? What factors impact your client's judgment? Is he or she impulsive? Does your client think only about the present moment or have the ability to think about the future (and how current actions might impact the future)? Is your client easily influenced by others or able to resist peer pressure? Does he or she learn from past mistakes, which can help one develop better judgment?

Understanding of Others

How capable is your client of understanding others, and of showing empathy for them? Is he or she able to see things from another person's point of view? Is your client able to read social cues, such as how another person may be feeling? How tolerant or accepting of differences is your client?

Self-Esteem

Does the child or adolescent have good self-esteem? Are your clients able to identify their strengths? What kinds of successes or accomplishments have they had? What do they feel are their shortcomings? In what areas do your clients feel insecure? Some key areas where children or adolescents may have insecurities include academic abilities or intelligence, athletic ability, fitting in socially, and body image.

Temperament

Assessing temperament or personality can help you better understand a child's or adolescent's behavior or mood. For example, temperament may explain why some children maintain a cheerful disposition while others are prone to negativity. Temperament may also be a factor in why some children are easier to parent than others. Parents can experience frustration if they fail to recognize how temperamentally difficult some things may be for their child to do. Children who struggle making transitions can become resistant and easily frustrated when asked to move quickly from one activity to another.

In *The Difficult Child*, Turecki and Tonner (2000) suggest 10 traits to consider when evaluating a child's or adolescent's temperament:

1. How active or restless is the child generally?
2. Does the child exercise good self-control or is he impulsive?
3. Is the child easily distracted or can she maintain focus or attention?
4. How intense is the child (e.g., loud, forceful personality, dramatic)?
5. How predictable is the child's physiological functioning (sleep patterns, appetite, etc.)?
6. Once the child is involved in something, can she stay with it a long time (positive persistence)? Conversely, how stubborn is she when she wants something (negative persistence)?
7. Does the child get easily overwhelmed by sensory stimuli such as loud noises, bright lights, strong smells, the taste or texture of foods, pain, or the texture of clothing?
8. What is the child's initial response to new situations (e.g., new experiences, places, or people)? Does he approach or withdraw?
9. How easily does the child adapt to change or transitions?
10. Is the child's predominant mood sunny or more serious?

Peers

Peers are generally an important part of life for a child, particularly as they grow older and become adolescents. A number of factors need to be considered when assessing peers. First, what does your client's circle of friends look like? Does it include one or more close friends, or is he or she isolated? If the individual has few or no friends, why is that? Does it reflect a deficit in social skills? What types of friends does the child or adolescent have? This will help you determine what type of influence peers might have on your client. Do the peers drink or use drugs? Is your client involved in a gang? Conversely, is he or she involved in any prosocial groups, such as a youth group at church or school groups? How much peer pressure does your client experience from these groups?

Second, is the individual having problems with any peers? Does he or she frequently get into fights with others? Is your client being bullied or picked on by anyone? If so, is it by one or several individuals? Why does your client think he or she is being bullied or picked on?

Third, you will want to explore dating with adolescents. Are they actively dating? If so, do they currently have a boyfriend or girlfriend? If so, how do they feel about the relationship? Is the boyfriend or girlfriend of a similar age? If your client is not dating, what are the reasons for not doing so? Does the teen have insecurities in regard to dating?

For adolescents who are dating, you will want to determine if they are sexually active. If so, what type of behaviors do they engage in? Are they practicing safe sex? Do they have any concerns in regard to sex or sexual orientation? Most teens will not volunteer their questions or concerns. The therapist has to ask. In addition, the therapist has to ask in a way that communicates, "I'm comfortable with this topic and you can be also. This is a safe place to discuss your questions or concerns."

Emotions

There are different dimensions of a child's or an adolescent's emotional life that should be explored. First, what is the general mood of the client? Does he or she generally maintain a positive mood or show signs of being depressed, such as sadness, irritability, or withdrawal? Does the child or adolescent generally appear confident, or is he or she often anxious? What is behind the depressed mood? Is there any evidence that your client may be suicidal? What situations make your client feel anxious? Young children, for example, may have fears about separation from their parents or loved ones.

Second, you should assess the child's or adolescent's ability to regulate emotions. How often does the client become angry, and what does this look like? Does your client calm or soothe him- or herself when upset, or remain flooded or upset for a long period of time? Does the child or adolescent ever threaten to harm him- or herself, or perhaps others, when upset?

Third, it can be helpful to assess what factors impact the child's or adolescent's mood. Is he or she getting sufficient rest on a consistent basis? Some parents do not set an appropriate bedtime for children or are inconsistent in what time children are put to bed. Tiredness or fatigue can cause or exacerbate a child's problems regulating his or her mood. Does the child become frustrated doing certain activities? Children with a learning disability or other academic difficulties may become frustrated or resistant around homework. As discussed earlier, temperament may be another factor that impacts your client's mood.

Outside Interests

Soliciting information regarding outside interests can be important in working with children and adolescents in a number of ways. If your client is a reluctant participant in therapy, discussing an outside interest can facilitate joining. Many adolescents appreciate a therapist who takes an interest in a topic that is important them. Adolescents, for example, can be invited to bring in music that is meaningful to them and discuss how the lyrics reflect what is going on in their lives.

Exploring outside interests can also give you a window into what is important to your client. Outside interests may reflect what your client feels passionate about. Examining outside interests can be a springboard for discussing issues around identity and meaning, themes that are important for many adolescents. Exploring your client's activities may also help you uncover client strengths, since individuals like activities that use their talents. Jonathan, who frequently engaged in graffiti, felt it showcased his artistic ability.

It can also be helpful to assess the breadth of your client's activities, as well as the time spent on the activities. Some children spend hours playing video games at the expense of schoolwork and chores, or instead of interacting with others. Other children may be overbooked with numerous activities (e.g., sports, music lessons, part-time jobs), creating stress because they have little downtime. Overscheduling of activities could also make it difficult for children or adolescents to devote enough time to their studies, impacting grades.

Psychopathology

When interviewing children or adolescents, you should be alert to possible signs of mental illness or substance abuse. The next chapter focuses on common mental disorders in children and adolescents, and how to assess for them.

Loved Ones

In addition to peers, it is important to assess the child's or adolescent's perspective on family and other loved ones. Exploration in this area should address both whom the youth considers important within the family and the quality of these relationships.

You should first examine who is in the caretaking role for your client. Does he or she live with one or both parents, or is someone else in the parenting role (e.g., grandparents, aunts or uncles, foster parents)? If your client is not living with his or her parents, how did this come to be? If raised by someone other than the parents, what role does the child or adolescent view the caregiver as having? Ali was adopted as a 1-year-old by her maternal grandparents. Therefore, she referred to her grandparents as Mom and Dad since this was the role they played in her life when she was growing up. Similar issues may arise in stepfamilies. Children raised by a stepparent from an early age may view the stepparent as Mom or Dad, particularly if they have little or no contact with one of the biological parents. In contrast, older children or adolescents may reject any parenting role for a stepparent.

You should also assess what kind of relationship the child or adolescent has with each parent, stepparent, or caregiver. Is it close or distant? Is it conflictual? Is there any evidence of neglect or abuse? Are there any signs of attachment issues? If a parent does not live with the child or adolescent, what kind of contact or relationship, if any, does the client have with this parent? If there is minimal or no relationship, does the child or adolescent feel angry, rejected, or distressed by this?

You should also inquire if your client has any brothers or sisters, since siblings can play an important role in a person's life. If your client has siblings, what kind of relationship do they have? Are they close? How much conflict exists between siblings? For older children and adolescents, you should explore if they are responsible for the care of younger siblings, perhaps even in a parentified role. Conversely, does your client have an older sibling who plays an important caretaking role? Also inquire as to how well other siblings are doing. It is not uncommon for other children to experience difficulties if family dynamics are problematic.

You should also explore whether there are other extended family members (e.g., grandparents, aunts, uncles, cousins) who are important to your client. Do any of these family members live with your client? What role or relationship do they have with the child or adolescent? In some families, grandparents may play an important caregiving role in addition to that provided by the parents.

Assessing loved ones will overlap with family assessment, discussed in Chapters 9 and 10. You will learn a lot about a child's or adolescent's functioning while conducting a family assessment. Conversely, family dynamics may be uncovered when assessing the child or adolescent. Attachment issues should lead you to carefully explore the type of parenting the child is receiving. Are they explained by a history of abuse or neglect? We firmly believe that any assessment of children and adolescents should be done in conjunction with an assessment of the family system. A failure to include the family in your assessment risks overlooking critical or important contextual variables in your client's life.

Education or Academics

One of the strongest motivators for parents to seek advice from a mental health specialist is concern about their child's academic performance. Most parents have high hopes for their children's academic and professional success. Thus, poor school performance worries parents. In addition, schools often refer children for evaluations when they are concerned about behavior, academic progress, or social problems.

You should ask a number of different questions when exploring education or academics. How is the child doing in terms of grades? If your client is struggling with low grades, is it in all classes, or is it in specific classes? Has he or she had a long history of academic difficulties, or is it a more recent problem? If it has a recent onset, have any changes occurred that coincide with the decline in academic performance? This might include changes at school (e.g., different teachers, new school), changes at home (e.g., separation or divorce, stressful life event), or beginning to use drugs.

It is also important to assess if there are any concerns around behavior or conduct at school. Have these concerns recently emerged, or is there a history of behavioral issues? Answers to these questions may give you some important clues as to possible psychopathology. ADHD, for example, may manifest early as a difficulty staying on task or in one's seat, or taking turns with classmates.

If there is any evidence of problems at school, then one should consider talking to the teacher, and perhaps even doing an observation at the school. Obviously teachers are in the best position to convey how the child is doing academically. They may even be aware of possible signs that suggest some type of learning disability or processing difficulty. Teachers can also offer important insights into how a child interacts with peers.

Learning disabilities or other processing difficulties should be ruled out in children or adolescents with a history of academic problems. If a learning disorder is suspected, then a referral for psychological testing should be made. As an advocate for the children you treat, you should know about the resources in your community.

Who are the qualified child specialists who can conduct a thorough evaluation? Developmental-behavioral pediatricians are specially trained to help children with learning problems. In addition, developmental psychologists and neuropsychologists also have specialized training in children's disorders. If possible, find out if your client has access to one of these child specialists. Ideally, an interdisciplinary team will evaluate the child or adolescent to provide a comprehensive assessment. The team might also include educators, family therapists, occupational therapists, speech therapists, child psychiatrists, and other professionals who work with children.

Unfortunately, learning evaluations can be costly and time consuming. Parents may not have the resources to help their children. Hopefully, the children you treat can, at a minimum, receive an educational evaluation through the schools.

In general, psychological testing assesses several learning categories, including IQ (intelligence), attention, memory, learning, visual perception and visual motor skills, and executive functioning. The latter refers to the ability to make decisions, plan, and execute—like a good executive secretary. Also, testing usually includes educational and achievement tests that might evaluate reading comprehension, vocabulary, spelling, math, writing, and language and speech skills. If a significant gap exists between a child's potential (as measured by tests of innate ability) and performance (as measured by academic and achievement tests), the child might be diagnosed with a learning disability.

A thorough evaluation includes ruling out other causes for learning problems, such as an undetected vision or hearing problem. A multidisciplinary team (i.e., a neuropsychologist, pediatrician, and other professionals) can provide the most comprehensive assessment. Some assessments include evaluation of behavior, social skills, development, emotions, and other measures. Evaluators also want histories of the child's learning and development, as well as an understanding of the child's current social world. Ideally, the therapist, teacher, and the parents can articulate specific questions based on observations that help guide the assessment.

Once the evaluation is done, parents are usually given a report that documents the child's strengths and weaknesses. Often, these reports are confusing because they assume a level of technical knowledge that most parents don't have. For those wanting to learn more about psychological testing, Braaten and Felopulos (2004) describe common questions and tests that are included in an evaluation in their book *Straight Talk about Psychological Testing for Kids*. Faraone's (2003) book *Straight Talk about Your Child's Mental Health* is another excellent resource for parents. In addition, Levine's *A Mind at a Time* (2002) and *The Myth of Laziness* (2003) offer explanations about learning challenges children can face.

If the school did the testing, adults involved with the child often meet to discuss the results and what changes might help the child. Many of the suggestions for amelioration of the child's weaknesses depend on adults in the child's life creating a new and different environment. Thus, even with a comprehensive evaluation, the child may not improve if the suggestions in the report are not implemented.

CASE EXAMPLES USING THE *JUST PEOPLE* MNEMONIC

The following case examples illustrate how the JUST PEOPLE mnemonic can be helpful in evaluating child or adolescent functioning. The first example illustrates its application with a preadolescent girl, and the second with an adolescent male.

Case Example of Selena

A therapist brought in for supervision the case of Selena, who had been referred to therapy by a nurse practitioner. Selena was a Hispanic girl (age 11) who had encopresis and incontinence as the presenting issues. The young girl had been hospitalized three times due to severe constipation, with the most recent hospitalization being 7 months prior.

Selena lived with her maternal aunt along with her older brother. Selena's father lived in another country, while her mother had passed away 18 months earlier. Selena began living with her aunt approximately 5 years ago after she and her brother were removed from the mother's home due to neglect and substance abuse.

The therapist presenting the case expressed confusion as to what to work on in therapy. The therapist had considerable information about Selena, enabling the supervisor and therapist to evaluate the client in the areas covered by JUST PEOPLE. There did not appear to be any concerns about Selena's *judgment*, which seemed appropriately mature for her age. Selena was a caring child, reflecting her ability to be empathic or *understand others*. She also seemed to have an appropriately healthy *self-esteem*, easily able to identify strengths or things she liked about herself. In terms of *temperament*, Selena was generally perceived as an easy child to parent. Both the aunt and the therapist noted that Selena generally maintained a positive mood, which may have been partly due to her temperament. Although Selena was a bit reserved when dealing with new situations, taking a little time to warm up, it did not seem to be an impairment.

Selena was doing well with *peers* since she had multiple friends, including one best friend. In terms of *emotions*, Selena was generally a happy person. Selena admitted being occasionally sad at the loss of her mother and recent death of her grandfather, but these feelings seemed appropriate given the loss of these two important figures in her life. Selena had *outside interests* that she enjoyed, such as art and nature walks. There did not appear to be any indications of *psychopathology*. The only concern the aunt had had was that Selena kept her room a bit messy. The therapist admitted to struggling with giving Selena a diagnosis, even though it was required as part of the treatment plan at her agency. Assessment of *loved ones* revealed Selena had a close relationship with her aunt, whom the therapist perceived to be a capable caregiver based on her observations. Selena also had a positive relationship with her brother. Finally, an assessment of her *educational* performance revealed that her grades were good (A's and B's) and that she had received good marks in citizenship for classroom behavior.

Based on assessment of the areas covered by JUST PEOPLE, Selena was functioning well, which explained why the therapist was having a difficult time figuring out what to do in therapy. Thus, it did not appear that the client needed therapy, and the encopresis was likely due to biological rather than psychological problems. Indeed, it was discovered that two biological relatives (biological mother and maternal grandfather) suffered from similar problems. Selena seemed to responding well to a new medication, and reported no longer having accidents.

Case Example of Sean

Sean is a 17-year-old Caucasian young man who has problems with his anger. He is easily irritated and short tempered. He has a history of fighting and was referred to counseling after getting into a fight at school. He said that he was helping out a friend who was being "hassled by some guy on the football team." He was suspended for fighting and warned he would be expelled if another incident occurred. He wasn't overly concerned about this.

His mother has been married three times and has been separated from her current husband for about 6 months. Sean reports that his mother was abused both by his father and her second husband. He says he is now big enough to make sure that it won't happen again. He denies ever being physically abused. There are no other children in the home.

The therapist uses the JUST PEOPLE mnemonic to guide his initial assessment of Sean. The therapist discovers that Sean's *judgment* is hampered by his impulsivity. He tends to react quickly to situations and fails to consider the consequences of his behavior. He seems to have trouble learning from his past mistakes, as he continues to repeat the same behavior. He gets in fights, most of the time to protect others. While his intentions are positive, his poor impulse control gets him into difficult situations. He reports showing good judgment in response to his drug and alcohol use. Sean says he has not used drugs, but occasionally drinks with friends on the weekends. He's had one incident where he came home drunk and his mother took away his truck. He says he knows better than to drink and drive.

Sean's *understanding of others* is evident in his empathy for friends, particularly when he sees they are in need of help. He has functioned in a protector role both at home with his mother and his friends.

When asked to identify his strengths, Sean initially struggles to answer the question, indicating possible issues with *self-esteem*. After some thought, Sean states his strengths are limited to his musical abilities. Another indication of Sean's low self-esteem is his lack of concern regarding the possibility of being expelled from school. It is as if he doesn't really care what happens to him.

In terms of *temperament*, Sean seems to struggle with self-control as evidenced by his impulsivity. Despite his impulsivity, Sean does show some ability to concentrate on things, particularly things that he enjoys such as music. He will also invest time in playing the drums, demonstrating positive persistence when learning things that interest him. His persistence, however, is also evident in being stubborn at times. Sean seems to have a serious and somewhat pessimistic mood, something that he always remembers having, even as a child.

Sean has some difficulty with *peers*. His friends tend to be younger than he is and he often takes on the role of their protector. He doesn't have a best friend and has never had a girlfriend. When asked about girls, he says he doesn't have enough time for that. He admits he can be hard to get along with "'cause I like things my way. Sometimes it is easier just to be alone." While he loves playing the drums, he has had some difficulty getting along with his band members. "I keep having to switch groups. I can't seem to find the right one."

In terms of *emotions*, Sean is struggling. He has had anger problems since he was very young. This may be due, in part, to having witnessed physical and verbal abuse at home from an early age. He can easily become angry and irritated with very little provocation. He is not aware of much in the way of feelings beyond anger.

Music is Sean's primary *outside interest*. Sean plays the drums in a band. He is passionate about music and hopes to continue playing professionally. He also feels some sense of admiration from other people in regard to his musical talent. Sean works after school delivering pizzas and shows some stability and responsibility in holding his part-time job.

After the initial assessment, the therapist has some possible ruleouts in terms of *psychopathology*. The therapist wonders if Sean may be depressed as evidenced by his irritability, low self-esteem, and pessimistic view of the world. There is also some concern about Sean developing a conduct disorder, although the therapist views this as less likely. His difficulty with peers is of concern but doesn't appear pathological.

Sean's primary *loved one* is his mother. He reports that they are very close and he feels very protective of her. He has little communication with his father. He has been close with his grandparents on his mother's side and feels very supported by them. His grandfather took him camping and fishing when he was younger but lately they haven't been able to find the time.

The primary concern regarding *education* is that Sean is in danger of being expelled from school due to his fighting. Sean is average in terms of academic performance, getting mostly B's and C's. Further assessment of other factors, such as his level of motivation and educational goals, is needed.

By using JUST PEOPLE, the therapist was able to identify areas where Sean was struggling as well as his strengths. Although further assessment is warranted in many areas, the therapist has an excellent starting point for understanding the client's functioning.

ASSESSMENT INSTRUMENTS FOR CHILDREN AND ADOLESCENTS

A variety of available instruments for assessing children and adolescents can supplement clinical interviewing and observation. The most widely used instruments for general assessment are those developed by Conners and Achenbach. The Conners Comprehensive Behavior Rating Scales (CBRS) are intended for youth between the ages of 6 and 18, and include a parent form, teacher report form, and a youth self-report form (Conners, 2008). Conners Early Childhood is available for assessing children ages 2–6 (Conners, 2009). Like the Conners scales, the Achenbach System of Empirically Based Assessment (Achenbach & McConaughy, 2003) includes forms that are completed by parents (Child Behavior Checklist), teachers (Teacher Report Form), and the child or adolescent (Youth Self-Report). The Child Behavior Checklist exists in two versions, one for children 6–18 and another for children 1½–5. There is also the Caregiver–Teacher report form for day care or preschool teachers to complete for children ages 1½–5.

Other systems for assessing children and adolescents include the Behavior Assessment System for Children (BASC). Like the scales described above, the BASC includes forms that can be completed by parents, teachers, and the child or adolescent (Thorpe, Kamphaus, & Reynolds, 2003). Another alternative is a family of scales (Lachar & Gruber, 2003) that consists of the Personality Inventory for Children, 2nd edition (parent report), the Personality Inventory for Youth (self-report), and the Student Behavior Survey (teacher report).

All of these scales are helpful in assessing whether the child's or adolescent's behavior or functioning is in the normative or non-normative range. Thus, these instruments can be particularly helpful in screening for possible disorders. Instruments intended to assess specific disorders in children and adolescents are discussed in the next chapter.

CONCLUSION

This chapter has highlighted the ways in which assessing children and adolescents differs from assessing adults. Understanding developmental issues is critical in assessing children and adolescents. It informs both what information needs to be assessed and how the information is collected. Assessment with a young child and an adolescent may be significantly different due to the developmental differences between the two.

Despite these differences, there is some overlap between assessing children and adolescents in terms of their functioning. The JUST PEOPLE mnemonic can help you recall the important areas of functioning to assess for children and adolescents. It can be used to identify both strengths and areas of concerns. To aid you in assessing for possible psychopathology, the next chapter focuses on common mental health disorders among children and adolescents.

CHAPTER 8

Assessing for Psychopathology in Children and Adolescents

As mentioned in the earlier chapter on assessing adults, you should note signs (observable behaviors or traits) and symptoms (concerns or complaints articulated by the child and the family) when assessing a child. This will help you identify syndromes which entail, "symptoms, signs and events that occur in a particular pattern and indicate the existence of a disorder" (Morrision, 2007, p. 11).

Being able to recognize DSM syndromes without becoming exclusively focused on a specific syndrome can be challenging. Frequently, new therapists are strongly influenced by their professional environments as they decide how much to focus on DSM diagnoses. If they are in a setting that stresses using DSM labels, student therapists will usually adopt the same perspective. If, on the other hand, they work in clinics that focus more on development, narrative, or environment, students might not think about DSM diagnoses at all.

Another challenge is discerning the presence of a diagnosable syndrome when the caretakers in the child's life describe different concerns. For example, the school or parents might complain about a child's behavior and look to the therapist to "fix the child." As long as the disruptive behaviors abate, the adults in the child's life might be satisfied. Nevertheless, treatment might be incomplete.

The age of the child also influences the therapist's ability to identify a known syndrome. The therapist might have a challenging time discriminating between normal developmental variations and psychopathology. In general, the younger the child, the more challenging it is to obtain an accurate diagnosis.

In addition, the therapist needs to consider whether treatment is necessary and what kinds of treatment might work. Again, the age of the child strongly influences these decisions. While the DSM diagnosis may pertain to the child, both the forces that perpetuate the problems and the means of amelioration may be beyond the child's control. In general, the younger the child, the more the treatment should be directed at parenting and the home environment.

Given all these considerations, a therapist must listen to the child and his or her caretakers and simultaneously maintain an inquisitive stance. A therapist might consider the following general assessment questions:

- Does the child have a known clinical syndrome (the only DSM question)?
- What is the etiology of the problem? Does it matter in terms of treatment planning?
- What forces maintain the problem?
- Are there other problems such as a physical health problem (diabetes), a family problem (divorce), or a learning problem (reading disorder) that influence the child's diagnosis (depression)?
- What forces support the child's strengths and healing?
- How are the family and the school influencing the child's struggles?
- What normal developmental issues does the child face, and how is the problem affecting his or her development?
- Is treatment necessary? How intense should the treatment be (multimodal methods, frequency of treatment, outside referrals, etc.)?
- What type of interventions will be most helpful and safe, and support the child's natural strengths and development?

To illustrate a biopsychosocial view of children's assessment, Table 8.1 outlines the problems/strengths list for three children. A therapist working with Johnny, Amanda, or Wayne would be remiss

TABLE 8.1. Problem and Strengths List for Three Children

Johnny, age 14	Amanda, age 9	Wayne, age 5
DSM diagnoses • ADHD (inattentive type) • Phobias (needles, spiders) • Social phobia *Physical diagnoses* • Irritable bowel syndrome *Environmental stressors* • Parents' divorce • Bullied at school *Strengths and resources* • Committed parents • Strong athlete	*DSM diagnoses* • Panic attacks • Depression (?) *Physical diagnosis* • Type I diabetes *Developmental issues* • Struggles separating from mother *Learning challenges* • Reading disorder • Working memory weakness *Environmental stressors* • Poverty • Older brother in prison *Strengths and resources* • Caring teacher • Supportive grandparents • Strong social skills	*DSM diagnoses* • ADHD? *Physical diagnosis* • Asthma *Developmental issues* • Night terrors *Environmental stressors* • Single parent with depression • Frequent moves *Strengths and resources* • Caring primary care doctor • Good day care

if he or she focused exclusively on the child's DSM diagnosis. In fact, other issues may impede effective treatment. For example, if Wayne's mother decides to move out of state with her boyfriend, the therapist will not be able to help Wayne. If Amanda continues to feel ashamed at school because of her poor academic performance and worried about her family's safety, it may be difficult to treat her panic and depression. If Johnny's uncontrolled diarrhea, which is caused by his irritable bowel, worsens, it may be unrealistic to think that the therapist can effectively treat his social phobia. Thus, while the therapists might accurately diagnose DSM disorders, their assessments are incomplete and will not lead to effective treatment if they don't consider holistic views of their clients.

Below are some questions to consider when evaluating a child for some of the most common DSM disorders. Clusters of positive answers to some of these questions might lead the therapist to read more about a specific diagnosis. One could read more detailed descriptions while maintaining a cautious skepticism about the accuracy of some sources, especially on the Internet. In addition, a therapist can purchase a copy of the DSM and have it as a ready reference when questions emerge. Consulting with your supervisor or another experienced therapist who has seen the variations of childhood disorders can help you identify significant signs and symptoms. If you are a beginning therapist, we caution you to be conservative in your diagnostic assessments. Giving a diagnosis to a child or adolescent is a serious responsibility. Turn to your supervisor and other more experienced therapists if you are unsure about the accuracy or utility of making a specific diagnosis.

BEHAVIOR DISORDERS IN CHILDREN AND ADOLESCENTS

In recent years, child specialists have focused increasingly on children's ability to regulate their emotions. One reason for this focus is that neuroscience research has identified specific parts of the brain that are the centers for skills like emotion regulation. For example, the prefrontal cortex and the amygdala are both important sources of emotion regulation. Child specialists have also noted that boys struggle with impulsive emotion regulation more often than girls. In contrast, girls struggle more with internalizing painful emotions such as sadness and worry. Thus, boys' emotional struggles may be more readily identifiable than girls' because boys are more likely to disrupt their environment—at school or at home. There are three primary diagnoses under the broad category of behavior disorders: attention-deficit/hyperactivity disorder (ADHD), oppositional defiant disorder (ODD), and conduct disorder (CD). In addition, future additions to the DSM[1] might include temper dysregulation disorder with dysphoria, a diagnosis that describes children who are moody, anxious, and irritable (Roan, 2010)

Attention-Deficit/Hyperactivity Disorder

ADHD can be characterized by three primary symptoms: inattention, hyperactivity, and impulsivity. It is one of the most common childhood diagnoses, occurring in up to 10% of children. It is more common in boys than girls, and the symptoms must be present before the child is 7 years old. In addition, children with ADHD often have other disor-

---

[1] Proposed changes for DSM-5 can be viewed at *www.dsm5.org.*

ders such as anxiety, depression, learning disorders, and other behavior disorders. Recently, some ADHD researchers have focused on emotion dysregulation as a core symptom and perhaps the underlying process of the other three symptoms (Barkley, 2005; Mash & Barkley, 2007).

ADHD is both overdiagnosed and underdiagnosed. Parents may be reluctant to consider a diagnosis of ADHD because they have read about its misuse in the press. In addition, ADHD can take many forms, so one child with ADHD might look very different from another. For example, some children, especially girls, are never hyperactive. Instead, teachers and parents consider them to be "daydreamers" and "unfocused." This form of ADHD is in fact called "inattentive type" because the child is "spacey," not overactive. Another reason ADHD can be so confusing is that the core symptoms often change as a child ages. Many children with ADHD outgrow their hyperactive symptoms, but the other core symptoms such as inattention and disorganization remain into adulthood. Other children seem to entirely outgrow their ADHD symptoms.

If you suspect that a child has ADHD or one of its subtypes, you should help the parents obtain a thoughtful professional evaluation of their child. Children and adults with ADHD face a host of challenges. They may struggle with schoolwork, job challenges, relationships, poor driving, or substance abuse. It is unfortunate that some children with ADHD are never diagnosed because excellent treatments for ADHD exist. Both medications and behavioral therapies have been shown to transform children's lives. In contrast, undiagnosed ADHD can lead to a life of personal failures.

Assessment of ADHD can be done by a pediatrician or an expert in child development. In addition, many school psychologists have the skills to accurately diagnosis ADHD in students. A neuropsychological assessment can also provide an accurate diagnosis. Since ADHD is one of the most common disorders of childhood, you should consider it whenever you see children who struggle with controlling their emotions and behavior. ADHD robs children of a key ingredient for success in life—focused attention. Thus, accurately identifying this common disorder can change the trajectory of a child's life.

Oppositional Defiant Disorder

ODD is characterized by the following symptoms: stubborn, argumentative, and disobedient. Like ADHD, this disorder is common and occurs more frequently in boys than girls. Children with ADHD are frequently also diagnosed with ODD, and sometimes ODD can lead to Conduct Disorder. To be diagnosed with ODD, a child must exhibit the signs and symptoms in several settings, although parents usually report that the child is worse at home than in other settings.

If the child's behavior moves from irritating to cruel and even sadistic, ODD is not an accurate diagnosis. Instead, the child with ODD can be characterized as argumentative, angry, defiant, spiteful, and annoying. Many children could appear to have ODD at some point in their lives. Thus, some mental health professionals question the usefulness of this diagnosis. Perhaps the utility of identifying this cluster of symptoms is that it can reveal some potentially serious problems. Symptoms of ODD may indicate that the child is depressed, especially if the main symptom is irritability. Also, the child may both be depressed and have ODD.

In addition, ODD behaviors seldom occur in isolation. Often, a child with ODD has siblings with similar struggles or parents who have difficulty providing the child with a warm, structured, nurturing environment. Fathers may be in jail, mothers may be depressed, and siblings may be in trouble with authorities or have substance abuse problems. The earlier these family problems appear in the family or the earlier the child displays ODD symptoms, the worse the prognosis. For example, Andy's mother was depressed when he was born and for the first few years of his life. His father was seldom home, and when he was home, Andy's parents would argue and even become violent. Andy's older brother, who was in high school, was already in trouble with the law because of his drug use. Thus, in his chaotic home environment, Andy's needs were virtually ignored until he got into a fight at school. In this scenario, focusing exclusively on Andy's "disorder" would be woefully inadequate.

Several variables predict that ODD can be a harbinger of further chaos and destruction. If the child uses drugs or alcohol, the prognosis is worse. More serious symptoms at earlier ages, such as violent behavior before age 9 or 10, also predict worse outcomes. The level of dysfunction in the child's family also influences the possibilities of effective treatment.

Evaluating any problems of children and teens should include an environmental assessment, especially evaluating the family (Gottman, DeClaire & Siegel, 1997). Indeed, family assessment is paramount in ODD since ODD is a diagnosis focused on family inter-action. DSM-IV-TR (American Psychiatric Association, 2000) notes that "there may be a vicious cycle in which the parent and child bring out the worst in each other. Oppositional Defiant Disorder is more prevalent in families in which childcare is disrupted by a succession of different caregivers or in families in which harsh, inconsistent, or neglectful child-rearing practices are common. . . . [ODD] is more common in families in which there is serious marital discord" (pp. 100–101).

Conduct Disorder

CD is a step beyond ODD in terms of dangerous behaviors. Symptoms of CD include a persistent pattern of behavior in which the basic rights of others or major social norms are violated. Children with CD destroy property, steal, and exploit and abuse other people. These children may be aggressive bullies, have frequent physical fights, use weapons, and be physically cruel to people or animals. Physical or sexual violence commonly occurs. The earlier these horrific behaviors begin, the worse the prognosis for the child. In fact, the DSM divides CD into types depending on the age of onset of the behaviors and their danger, severity, and cruelty. Children and teens are diagnosed with CD only up to age 18. Afterwards, the diagnosis would usually change to antisocial personality disorder.

Children and teens with CD have little empathy or concern for the feelings, wishes, or well-being of others, including friends and family members. In fact, the teen with CD often misinterprets other people's behaviors as threatening or hostile and, in turn, responds with increased aggression. Even if they harm a friend or family member, these young people may feel little remorse. Like teens with ODD, teens with CD often abuse substances, take dangerous risks, and have early sexual experiences and volatile interpersonal relationships. Teens with CD seldom assume responsibility for their choices or behaviors. Instead, they blame others for their difficult lives. Usually, by the time children or teens are diagnosed with CD, they are in serious trouble with the law or other authorities such as school or community leaders. Thus, accurate assessment and treatment usually involves a comprehensive team approach and often includes professionals from a variety of settings including school workers, legal professionals, therapists, and medical providers.

AFFECTIVE DISORDERS
IN CHILDREN AND ADOLESCENTS

Perhaps the most common diagnoses in children and adolescents are affective disorders, or disorders pertaining to emotions. Primary emotions that influence children and teens are sadness, fear, and worry. In addition, many depressed or anxious adults first developed symptoms of their affective disorders when they were young. In fact, many times these disorders started around age 11 or even earlier. While parents and other adults cling to the myth of the carefree days of childhood, this is often not reality for many children and teens. Biology (including temperament and genetics) and environment (poor parenting, poverty, bullying at school) conspire to make childhood a time of stress for many children, not a time of idyllic joy.

Unfortunately, most children and teens with mental health issues never receive any treatment, thanks to our myths about happy children, and the fact that they lack awareness of mental disorders and adequate language skills to explain how they feel. Similar to adults, many children improve spontaneously. But others move into adulthood resigned to living lives of sadness and stress because they believe that living with these negative emotions is normal. In fact, children and teens who remain untreated are less likely to ever seek treatment as adults because sadness and worry have become a way of life.

Mood Disorders

Children and teens are at a distinct disadvantage when it comes to describing their mood disorders. Frequently, they do not have the insight or vocabulary to describe what they are feeling, especially compared to adults. In addition, their sadness may not be readily observable and it may last longer than a typical depressed mood in an adult. Instead, they do poorly in school, have troubled relationships, and are often irritable and angry. Thus, it is easy for a therapist to miss the diagnosis when a child has a mood disorder. In addition, like other diagnoses in children and teens, depression in children may be casually disregarded when a child is called "lazy, unruly, defiant" or a host of other labels. Thus, as a therapist, you must dig a little deeper in your assessment, consider depression as a primary diagnosis because it is so common, and observe the child's behaviors and interactions carefully.

Core symptoms of depression include ongoing sadness, irritability, or anger in a child or teen. Depression can occur in up to 5% of children and teens and usually starts at an earlier age for boys than girls. Many children who are depressed are also anxious and they may have other disorders such as ADHD or behavior disorders. As with other disorders, substance abuse makes the depressed child's difficult life even worse. Since all children and teens feel down at times, it is important to decide if treatment is warranted. When making this decision, consider the following questions:

- Has the child's weight changed significantly?
- Have the child's sleep patterns changed?
- Does the child lack energy and complain of fatigue?
- Does the child have problems concentrating or describe feeling worthless or guilty?
- Does the child have suicidal thoughts?

In addition to considering these questions, which help you assess the severity of the child's symptoms, you can also consider the duration of the symptoms and how well the child is completing the tasks of daily living. Unfortunately, when children are depressed, their symptoms often continue for long periods of time, sometimes for their entire early lives. While they go through their daily routines, they are not prospering. Thus, you should consider depression as a diagnosis. At times, you might think that they have good reason to be depressed when you observe their chaotic, lonely lives and challenging circumstances neither you nor the child can control. The stress in their lives should prompt you to take their depression even more seriously, not less, even when you cannot change the child's environment. Some research suggests that one major depressive episode in childhood makes the probability of another episode more likely. The research also suggests that smaller life stressors can provoke a second episode of depression (Spencer, 2006). Thus, as with ADHD, identifying depression early and providing effective treatment can change the direction of a child's life.

Bipolar Disorder

In addition to a depressed or sad mood, some children and teens also have euphoric moods and extreme irritability. In fact, a child might start out with a chronic depressed mood that later develops into a euphoric mood. When a child presents with these symptoms, you want to consider the diagnosis of bipolar disorder. As with ADHD, if you are unfamiliar with bipolar disorder, you should turn quickly to your supervisor or other experienced consultant for help. Bipolar disorder is a serious, chronic illness, and this diagnosis should be given to a child only by an experienced clinician. In addition, treatment for bipolar disorder almost always involves psychotropic medications, even for children. Thus, obtaining the help of an experienced physician from the start can benefit you and your clients.

It wasn't until recently that mental health providers even recognized that children and teens could have bipolar disorder. In earlier years, parents and providers were at a loss to understand a child who was extremely giddy or silly, defiant, and had grandiose thoughts about his or her abilities. Another child with bipolar disorder might present quite differently. Parents might report that the child has violent outbursts of screaming, kicking, biting, or other violent behaviors that continue for long periods of time. Parents are at a loss for how to help these children, and the intensity of the symptoms may scare and exhaust them (Wozniak, 2006).

Bipolar disorder in children and teens shares the common symptom of emotion dysregulation with ADHD. Thus, differential diagnosis is a critical issue. In general, ADHD starts before age 7, while bipolar symptoms usually start later. Dramatic mood changes are the prominent symptom in bipolar disorder and may not be present at all in children with ADHD. Often, children or teens with bipolar disorder have a parent who has been diagnosed with the disorder. Teasing out the correct differential diagnosis can be challenging even for experienced clinicians. Thus, your initial responsibility, if you suspect that your client has bipolar disorder, may be making sure you guide your client to an experienced mental health provider who has assessed pediatric bipolar disorder many times.

Anxiety Disorders

Anxiety disorders are perhaps the most common disorders of childhood, especially when they are combined under one heading. Children and teens have many fears and worries, and there are many different categories of anxiety disorders (Hirshfeld-Becker & Geller, 2006). Social phobia, specific phobias, obsessive–compulsive disorder, separation anxiety, posttraumatic stress disorder, and generalized anxiety disorder are some of the most common childhood disorders. In our experience, the boundaries between these disorders are less rigid than those between other diagnoses. A child or teen with social phobia will often have several specific fears and may have many worries in general. In addition, anxiety frequently co-occurs with other disorders such as depression, ADHD, and others. Also, anxiety seems to run in families. Thus, fearful children often have worried, anxious parents.

Children, especially children with weak verbal skills, may have a hard time identifying their fears. Instead their fears are expressed in such behaviors as clinging, avoidance, or crying, or in physical complaints such as stomach pains, nausea, and vomiting. Children and teens who can express their fears may complain of thoughts they have of disasters happening during daily events. For example, a child may think that his father's plane is going to crash when he is on his business trip. Thus, thoughts, behaviors, and physical sensations all contribute to anxiety. Parents may be confused and flustered by their children's intense emotions. A child may avoid a friend's birthday party when she learns that there will be balloons at the party. Another child may disrupt the family camping trip and even refuse to go because of his fear of spiders. Another child may refuse to go to school because she is worried that somehow her mother will be killed or kidnapped while they are apart. Since childhood worries are common, one way of recognizing when treatment is necessary is to think about how long the child has had the fear, how terrified the child is, and how the fear affects the child's daily life. In what ways is the child or family limited by the fear?

While anxiety can be learned, evidence exists that there is often a biological component. Thus, anxious, shy, cautious children frequently grow up to be anxious adults. For anxiety disorders, early intervention—especially providing skills to help children conquer their fears—can help the children long after the actual treatment has ended. Skills like challenging one's fear, graded exposure, relaxation, and assertiveness can be learned by families. Rapee and colleagues (2008) have created an excellent book entitled *Helping Your Anxious Child* to help parents identify and treat their children's fears. There is also an accompanying website, *www.ceh.mq.edu.au/hyac.html*, so that parents have the tools they need to help themselves and their children.

One diagnosis under the broad heading of anxiety disorders that deserves special mention is obsessive–compulsive disorder (OCD), which often begins in childhood around ages 10–14. OCD is a disorder of intrusive and persistent thoughts and ritualized behaviors to try and control the thoughts. OCD occurs in about 5% of children, is more common in boys than girls, and is often comorbid with tics. OCD runs in families and has a strong genetic loading. Often, total cure is not possible but learning to manage stress, early interventions, effective medications, and behavioral therapy can help a child with OCD live a fairly normal life.

Adults will usually notice that a child with OCD needs to perform some elaborate rituals that often involve washing, counting, checking, or hoarding. For example, a boy with OCD will find himself tapping on a tree on the playground every day. Often children's obsessive thoughts will focus on fears of aggression or contamination. For example, a teenager with OCD will be afraid to touch the doorknob because he fears it is contaminated with germs. As children with OCD age, they may develop more elaborate fears with sexual or religious themes. Thus, in diagnosing a teen with OCD, it is important to not get caught up in the content of the fear and instead focus on the patterns of thoughts and ritualized behaviors.

SUBSTANCE ABUSE

In reading about the previous disorders, you might have noticed that substance abuse makes stress and mental illnesses worse. The single most common mistake therapists make about substance abuse is not asking about it. Instead, the therapist accepts the child's or parents' views of the problems. Unfortunately, most children and teenagers will not bring up their substance use unless you ask. Thus, regardless of the problems that you are investigating, you should ask about (1) smoking, (2) alcohol, (3) marijuana, and (4) use of any other drug—either prescribed or nonprescribed. It should be a routine part of your interview, and if possible, you should ask parents about this as well, not just the children or teens.

Often, children and teens will minimize the significance of their drug use and hope that you will minimize it too. Don't. Keep asking, gently, until you obtain a thorough history of your clients' drug use and a thorough understanding of their current use. Your clients may not give you the full story initially. But, as you win their trust and respect, you can ask again. Thus, obtaining an accurate understanding of a young client's drug use may take several sessions. Part of obtaining a careful history means that you also understand the forces influencing your clients' drug use. If their social network or parents use drugs and alcohol, they probably will also, and stopping may involve changing social networks. Many forces influence adolescents' drug and alcohol use. Thus, you and your clients may not agree that their substance use is a problem or needs to change. You may have more motivation to address the issue than your clients do. In addition, they may not see any connections between, say, treating their ADHD and their substance use.

Besides directly asking your clients about substance use, you have other possible sources of information. You can ask other family members, obtain medical or school records, and obtain laboratory findings such as blood and urine tests. In fact, many parents who are concerned about drug use require teens to take random urine tests, using kits that they buy at a drugstore. Regardless of your sources of information, try not to put your clients in a position where they want to hide information from you.

Substance abuse is comorbid (coexisting) with many other child and adolescent disorders. Researchers try to discern which came first, the mental health problem or the substance abuse. It may be important to understand whether the substance "caused" the mental health problem or the mental health problem served as an impetus for substance abuse. At times, the two problems are independent of each other. If your client has been using a substance, say marijuana, daily for many months, he will not know the impact of the marijuana on his life or other problems, nor will you. Thus, clinicians ask their clients to totally stop the substance for a period of time, in essence to get it out of the client's system and to obtain an accurate understanding of its impact.

Another challenge that you will probably have to address is client confidentiality. Therapists have many varied perspectives on what to keep private from parents or schools and what to share. They also have different views on when to share information and whether parents should be in charge of their teen's sobriety. The best way to address these issues systematically is to have a written description of your policies on confidentiality and to share them with the family during the initial session.

PERVASIVE DEVELOPMENTAL DISORDERS

Pervasive developmental disorders (PDDs) have received a lot of attention in the press. Specifically, autism has received attention from journalists and the federal government because of the increasing numbers of children diagnosed with autism. Many controversies surround autism, including disagreements about causes, rate of occurrence, and treatments. These controversies exist because little is known about autism and other PDDs including Asperger syndrome, childhood disintegrative disorder (CDD), and Rett syndrome.[2] What is known suggests that these disorders are frequently lifelong, with no cure, and that early diagnosis and intervention are critical for gains to be made. In general, children with PDD who have some language skills, higher intelligence, and some normal social interaction have a better prognosis. Also, medications that effectively treat these disorders do not exist. Thus, at this time, treatment focuses on symptom amelioration.

PDDs are a group of complex, chronic childhood disorders that cause multiple struggles including behavioral problems and trouble with communication and social skills. Often, infants appear to have normal development during the first few months of life, and only gradually do parents realize that some part of their child's development has gone awry. Specific struggles of children with PDD include impairment in "reciprocal social interaction skills, communication skills, or the presence of stereotyped behavior, interests, and activities" (American Psychiatric Association, 2000, p. 69). In recent years, research and public attention have been directed at ameliorating the symptoms of autism and Asperger syndrome.

Autism is a serious disorder that is more common in boys than girls. Children with autism have impaired social interaction and communication. In addition they have restricted repertoires of activities and interests. These children struggle with nonverbal behaviors such as eye contact and facial expressions. They often fail to develop friendships and struggle with skills such as emotional intelligence. Often, they are more interested in objects such as a computer than in people. The child's struggles are apparent early, before age 3. For some children, development will appear normal for the first few months of life and then the parents begin to note dramatic changes characterized by a gradual withdrawal from human interaction. Many, but not all, autistic children have low intelligence.

Asperger syndrome is also a disorder of serious and sustained impairment in social interaction with restricted, repetitive patterns of

---

[2] DSM-5 may combine the separate PDDs into a single disorder called autistic spectrum disorders, although this is being met with criticism (Roan, 2010).

behavior, interests, and activities. It is less common than autism, but like autism, it occurs more frequently in boys and starts at an early age. Children with Asperger syndrome have normal intelligence and do not have delays in language, thought, or self-help skills. Thus, they may do many of the normal activities of childhood, such as going to school, playing with friends, and playing video games. Challenges arise when they need to use strong language skills or show empathy for another child. Instead, these children shine when they need to learn details about a computer program or a scientific topic, or math skills. In addition, children with Asperger syndrome frequently have other disorders such as ADHD or tics. Since these disorders often create more social disruption, the symptoms of Asperger syndrome can be overlooked.

Autism and other PDDs present many challenges for families. Parents grieve as they watch their children fail to develop normally. As their child reaches each new developmental stage, the grief reoccurs as parents are reminded that their child is not following the trajectory of normal development. Parents wonder if they have somehow caused their child's struggles and what the future holds for their child. Often, children with PDD remain dependent on their parents, at least financially, for their entire lives. As parents face the reality of daily life with a child struggling with a PDD, they may feel angry and resentful. They may blame the child, their partner, or themselves.

We strongly recommend that you obtain a thorough developmental evaluation from an expert in PDD if you feel unqualified to make such a serious diagnosis. But, once the diagnosis is made, family therapists can offer the education and guidance that help sustain a family as the members seek ways to balance the needs of the child with PDD, the siblings, the parents, and the marriage. Many families report this balancing act is the toughest challenge they have ever faced.

EATING, SLEEPING, AND SEX

As you conduct your assessment of a child or teenager, consider the role of normal, daily physiological processes. For example, disrupted eating, sleeping, or sexual behavior can be a symptom of another disorder such as depression. Changes in physical functioning such as eating patterns can be disorders themselves, such as anorexia nervosa and bulimia. Finally, disrupted physical processes can be mediators that affect behavior and disorders. For example, many parents report that their children's ADHD symptoms are much worse in the evening when they are tired and hungry. Children who do not get enough sleep each night can easily develop "behavior disorders" that self-correct once the child has a daily routine that includes enough sleep and appropriate eating. While it is beyond the scope of this chapter to discuss each of these topics in detail, we encourage you to learn more about normal developmental processes and how they can go awry. In addition, identify some physician colleagues in your community whom you could use as resources when questions about these issues arise with your clients.

PARENTS OF CHILDREN WITH MENTAL DISORDERS

When working with children, in contrast to treating adults, you will be highly dependent on your "co-therapists"—the child's parents—for effective assessment and treatment. Historically, family therapy has focused on the family as the "symptom bearer." Individual diagnosis was often ignored by the early family therapists. Even worse, some early theories of psychopathology blamed parents for their child's mental health problems. According to some early theories, the "refrigerator mother" was so cold and distant that her child developed a mental illness.

Today, most mental health professionals are more interested in engaging the parents' help than in blaming them. As you begin your clinical work with children, you will quickly realize that the brief 50-minute weekly session is almost insignificant compared to the daily impact the parents have. The younger your client is, the more you must depend on his or her parents to accurately report the child's symptoms and, later, to carry out the treatment. In fact, some treatment programs for children have put the therapist in the role of consultant to the parents, who deliver the actual treatment to their children. Thus, the parents' ability to accurately report symptoms that improve or worsen over time and their motivation to help their children strongly influence the treatment outcomes.

As a family therapist, you will meet many different kinds of parents. Some parents want to drop their child off for treatment in the same way that they would take their car to the auto repair shop. Other parents are so overwhelmed with their own struggles—economic challenges, marital conflict, chronic illnesses—that even when they love their children deeply, they have little to offer. Still other parents may be so ashamed and full of guilt about their child's problems that they are virtually paralyzed. They have no ideas about how to help. Other parents are exhausted. They have tried everything they know to help their child. They are defeated and perhaps angry at the demands their child's problems have placed on their lives. Some parents may bring their children for treatment under duress. A school or another authority requires that the child get treatment. For divorcing parents, their children may be pawns in their ongoing marital conflict. For grieving or lonely parents, their children may unwittingly become their new "partners" and the child may become the parent to his or her parent.

Even if you believe a child or teen has a DSM disorder, individual treatment of that disorder will not be adequate. You must consider the parent's skills, energy, stressors, motivations, and attitudes when you conduct your assessment and plan treatment. In general, we remind our students that parents do not have to be perfect parents to ultimately help their children. If you can form an empathic relationship with the parents instead of covertly blaming them for their child's struggles, the assessment and treatment will be easier. Be careful to avoid falling into the trap of thinking that you are the child's protector who shields him or her from heartless, incompetent parents. At times, this might mean that you spend a session understanding the parents' lives and their struggles before you focus on the child. Usually, to be a competent child therapist, you must first be an empathic family therapist.

CONCLUSION

In recent years, therapists and researchers have acknowledged that in fact, many adult disorders start in childhood. Often, a child's symptoms go undetected or are attributed to "a phase" or "growing pains." However, accurately diagnosing a child and providing appropriate treatment early can prevent a lifetime of suffering. In addition, smaller interventions are often effective with children because their disorders have not yet become intractable. Thus, treating children and their families can be especially rewarding for therapists who recognize that their brief treatments might have changed the trajectory of their young clients' lives.

CHAPTER 9

Assessing Family Interaction

R egardless of who arrives in your office for the first appointment, it will be important to have a thorough understanding of family interaction and how it affects and is affected by the presenting problem. In order to do a thorough assessment of family interaction, it's ideal to have multiple family members present in the early stages of therapy. Because many clients view problems as "individual problems," your clients will either arrive at therapy alone or will bring a family member whom they think has a problem (e.g., a child with a behavior problem). You, the therapist, are the primary instrument in exploring family relationships and their connection to the presenting problem. As you'll see, family assessment is much more than simply gathering information about a family; it's a way to translate theoretical concepts into practice (Nichols & Everett, 1986).

Since we assume you have already been exposed to various theories for working with families, we are not going to use this chapter to cover each theoretical perspective on family assessment. Since different theories have different strengths, we believe it can be helpful to assess families from multiple perspectives. Therefore, the purpose of this chapter is to provide you with an integrative framework of diverse systemic concepts to assess and conceptualize family interaction in the here and now. In the next chapter, we describe assessment of the multigenerational family system, including transgenerational family patterns.

BARRIERS TO EFFECTIVE
FAMILY ASSESSMENT

Barrier 1: Therapist's Lack of Involvement in Scheduling the First Session

Family assessment begins with the first contact with your client. In some clinics, someone is designated as a phone intake person or there's a rotating schedule. A lack of involvement at this stage of client contact shields you from important information. Who calls to make the appointment? Who is mentioned (and not mentioned) in the description of the problem? The answers to these questions give you some initial impressions of the family relationships in your understanding of the presenting problem. For example, a mother may call about therapy for her daughter who is having behavioral problems at school. Such a presentation raises additional questions: Does her father live at home? Is he also concerned about problems at school? Are siblings present and are they having any difficulties? These are all questions that help create a context for the presenting concerns. They may not be answered in the first phone call, but they help establish an agenda for assessment during the first session. Another purpose of the first phone contact is deciding who will attend the first session.

Barrier 2: Not Including Multiple Family Members in the First Session and Beyond

Many beginning family therapists allow their clients to establish the structure of the therapy (Whitaker & Napier, 1978), such as the day, time, and, in some cases, the location of meetings. In addition, they allow their clients to decide who will attend sessions. We believe this is a mistake, for a variety of reasons, which we describe in another book (Patterson et al., 2009). In order to conduct a thorough family assessment, it's highly preferable that as many family members as possible attend the first session. Because many beginning therapists are intimidated by interviewing multiple family members, they're content to meet with the identified patient for all or part of the first session. Such a structure implicitly communicates agreement with the client's definition of the problem and severely limits a therapist's ability to assess the family. When multiple family members attend therapy, you're able to access multiple perspectives on the problem and see the family's interaction, rather than simply hearing one person's description of family relationships. For example, when a family is present you can collect data such as who sits next to whom, who talks first, who is quiet, and who talks for whom. When you wait to include family members later in treatment, your ability to see the problem systemically and help the family see the problem systemically becomes much more challenging. If you want multiple family members at the first session, you'll need to advocate for that position when scheduling the first appointment. We recognize that in some cases, regardless of your efforts, it won't be possible for multiple family members to attend due to a client's strong desire to be seen alone, the lack of availability of family members, or your own clinical judgment that including family members will be unproductive.

Barrier 3: Facilitating Dialogue between Client and Therapist, but Not between Family Members

Many young therapists are aware of the importance of getting the family members to talk to each other, but they feel anxious and out of control when family interaction gets going. Napier and Whitaker (1973) attribute the shutting down of family interaction to beginning therapists' overeagerness to help: "The family speaks a few sentences to each other, or speaks to [the therapist] about a family member, and the therapist is off—advising, commenting, questioning, interpreting, working" (p. 231). Of course, during the first session or two, the therapist will play a central role in questioning and data gathering. However, eventually you need to let the family expose their system to you, allowing you see them in action rather than just listening to a verbal description of something that happens elsewhere.

QUESTIONS TO BEGIN
FAMILY ASSESSMENT

One of the significant challenges our students face is how to inquire about the family. The family or individual client has described a problem and the students asks, "Now what do I do?" A common fear is that family members will be resistant to such questions and raise concerns that they're being blamed for the problem. It's certainly possible to offend families if they're asked the wrong questions, such as "Why don't you set better limits with your child?" Rather, our approach to family assessment emerges from the systems theory concept of "wholeness"—

each family member is impacted by experiences and by changes in another family member. With the concept of wholeness as a foundation, it becomes impossible *not* to inquire about family relationships.

Our first question when beginning a family assessment is "Who is in the family?" With the help of a genogram, which will be discussed in Chapter 10, you will want to identify all the family members. It's imperative that multiple family members participate in this discussion, because some family members will have different definitions of who is in the family and who isn't in the family. For example, a therapist was gathering family information from a couple who had been dating for 2 years. When the male partner finished identifying his siblings, his female partner interjected and asked about his sister, whom he hadn't included as a sibling. The male partner, embarrassed, acknowledged the omission, and told the story of his 2-year-old sister drowning when he was 9. He discovered her body in the pool and felt responsible for her death. Without his female partner's input, the therapist would have missed significant information.

Below are sample questions that help us continue an exploration of the family. They are not listed in any particular order, but rather as a menu of options.

> "What is your perspective on the problem?"
> "Who do you talk with about the problem?"
> "What have been the effects of the problem on the family?"
> "What is the sequence of events when the problem is present? (Who does what, when, where, and how?)"
> "Who is most concerned about this problem or person?"
> "Who else is aware of this problem?"
> "Who in the family isn't aware of the problem?"
> "Who has the most hope that this problem can be overcome? Who has the least hope?"
> "What do you believe caused or started the problem?" (Rolland, 1998)
> "How do you think other families cope with similar problems?" (Rolland, 1998)
> "Have there been any recent changes in family?"
> "What happens when the two of you (e.g., parents) talk with one another about your child's problem?"

"If grandmother were here, what would she say about this problem?"

"What have you tried to solve the problem?"

"What strengths and resources in the family can help you cope
with this problem?"

These questions elicit data about the family, whether family members
are present or not. The data that emerge from these questions can open
pathways to other relevant information and begins to inform your systemic assessment.

SYSTEMIC FAMILY ASSESSMENT

In addition to the data-gathering questions you're asking your clients
during the early stages of therapy, you also need to ask yourself a series
of reflective questions to organize the data and then place it in a systemic framework. By "systemic," we mean placing the problem in the
context of the family and considering the repetitive, circular patterns
of the family in its effort to cope with the problem. This reflective part
of your assessment provides emphasis and significance. In other words,
you're taking a wealth of data and organizing it into a cohesive summary using the language of systems theory. We've found that this systemic reflection is challenging for beginning therapists due to the smor-
gasbord of theoretical models (e.g., structural family therapy, Bowen
therapy, emotionally focused therapy), which may be easy to grasp on
paper but are difficult to put into practice. As mentioned earlier, rather
than attempting to offer family assessment guidelines from each theoretical model, we describe core assessment concepts that transcend specific theoretical models.

Circularity

When couples and families describe problems to us, they typically have
theories about causes of problems—"If she would stop nagging me all
the time, I would spend more time with her"; "The reason I yell at my
son is because he won't listen to me." Rarely do our clients provide
descriptions of problems that capture the contributions of multiple family members. Such "linear causality" is ingrained in American culture.
Therapists new to systemic thinking fall into similar traps of looking

for root causes of problems, which often keeps the focus on the identified patient.

An essential part of family assessment is looking for patterns of
interaction, which are usually repetitive and circular. Observing the
interactions of siblings provides a good example of circularity: Josh, age
7, is playing with his Legos, which he doesn't like to share. His brother
Brandon, age 9, tries to play with Josh but is rudely told to go away.
Feeling angry from the rejection, Brandon begins to tease Josh, which
leads to Josh getting frustrated and yelling at Brandon. Brandon likes
the attention and continues to tease Josh. Josh then gets up and starts
hitting Brandon. Brandon hits back and Josh starts to cry. Parents will
typically see the last part or none of this interaction, but will frequently
assign responsibility to one sibling. In this example, the mother and
father may view the problem differently based on their relationship with
and beliefs about each child and their own experiences (or lack of experience) as a sibling. Such circular and triangular (mother/father, Josh,
Brandon) patterns might repeat again and again. Rather than accepting
linear definitions of problems, such as that Brandon hit Josh and is a
bad kid, a key part of our assessment is exploring interactions around
problems, which helps make therapy with families a creative enterprise
(Nichols & Schwartz, 2007).

Subsystems, Hierarchy, and Boundaries

When assessing the family, it's helpful to visualize the system as a series
of three basic subsystems—the spousal, parent–child, and sibling subsystems. Each subsystem is both a whole and a part of other subsystems
and has its own unique culture, interactional roles, and hierarchy. Hierarchy defines the power structure of the family. It is useful to evaluate
who holds the power in the family and how it is demonstrated. Most
family therapists would endorse a hierarchy that grants shared power to
the parents, who have greater power than the children.[1] In many struggling families, the hierarchy will be poorly defined (unclear who has the
power in the family); rigidly defined (one or both parents give children
little, if any, power to make decisions); or incongruous (children have

---

[1] Of course, there are many caveats to this perspective. For example, in households that
include three or more generations, grandparents may play a significant caregiving role
due to parental absence and/or a cultural value of multigenerational parenting.

more power than the parents). Hierarchies exist in the family as a whole and in each subsystem. For example, you may observe that one partner has more power than the other partner in the spousal subsystem.

Power is generally seen overtly, such as when parents discipline their child for misbehavior or when a spouse overfunctions in the family and makes most of the major decisions. However, power can also be shown covertly. Covert power is seen through actions or behaviors and is often not readily apparent. If a child continually withdraws and does not respond to his parent's questions or comments, this can be a covertly powerful position. Passive–aggressive behavior can be very hard to predict and covertly powerful. It is often assumed that those in the family who speak the loudest are the most powerful. They may hold some overt power simply because they demand attention, but their power may be limited if they are ignored by other family members. In your assessment of subsystems and hierarchy in families, you'll want to ask yourself the following questions:

1. In which subsystem does the basic conflict (not necessarily the presenting problem) reside?
2. Is the current hierarchy functional for this particular family at this particular time?

In addition to subsystems and hierarchy, it will also be essential to assess boundaries in the family—internal boundaries between family subsystems and external boundaries between the family system and larger systems in the community (e.g., neighborhood, school, health care, legal). Boundaries are invisible lines that serve two primary purposes: (1) they define the membership of the family—who is in the family and who is outside the family; and (2) they regulate emotional and physical distance between subsystems and between family systems and the outside environment. You might want to think about boundaries on a continuum of permeability—from diffuse boundaries (high permeability) to closed boundaries (low permeability). A family with highly permeable internal boundaries may experience greater physical and emotional closeness, but little individual identity and autonomous functioning. In contrast, a family with impermeable internal boundaries will experience greater distance and autonomy, but little physical and emotional closeness.

Structural family therapists have written extensively about

enmeshed and disengaged families, which are regulated by boundaries. Enmeshed families have diffuse internal boundaries and closed external boundaries, which allows family members to intrude on each other's personal space and privacy and prevents or limits the entry of new information and individuals from the outside the family system (Walsh, 2006). Disengaged families have closed internal boundaries and diffuse external boundaries, which severely limits attachments and offers little protection from external intrusions and individuals (Nichols & Everett, 1986). Families will optimally define their boundaries as open or semipermeable, which would be at the center of the boundary continuum, allowing for necessary comfort and support while at the same time allowing each person enough freedom to express their age-appropriate autonomy.

Triangles

Within every family, you will see a variety of alignments between family members. As an experiment, think about your own family. It's likely that you can identify some dyads (e.g., mother–daughter, brother–sister) as close, while others are more distant or conflictual. If you examine those dyadic relationships in more detail and in the context of your whole family, you may notice that the distance or conflict in one or more dyads is associated with greater closeness in another dyad. For example, there may be conflict between an emotionally and physically distant husband and his wife, a close bond between the wife and their oldest daughter, and a distant relationship between the oldest daughter and her father. When the oldest daughter leaves the home, her younger sister takes on her role of Mom's confidant. Family therapists call this alignment a triangle: When a twosome experiences conflict, distance, and anxiety, pulling in a third person is an effort to cope with relational stress and stabilize the system (Guerin, Fogarty, Fay, & Kautto, 1996).

Triangles come in many different forms and arrangements. Two common family processes associated with triangles are parentification and scapegoating; both are the result of conflict and anxiety in the spousal subsystem. Parentification occurs when children are brought into the spousal subsystem to assume a highly responsible role in the care and well-being of the family, while also potentially tending to the emotional needs of a parent. Scapegoating occurs when a conflictual spousal subsystem turns its attention to a child's misbehavior to diffuse the stress in their troubled relationship. The scapegoated child is the classic identified patient: Parents will describe in laundry-list form the transgressions of the child while giving the impression that everyone else in the family is fine. In your assessment of families, you will want to recognize troublesome triangles.

Family Roles

In our description of triangles, we mentioned the family roles of parentified child and scapegoated child. These are just two of many roles in the family. Family roles are first identified as those that are prescribed, such as mother, father, son, or daughter. In assessing family roles it also useful to evaluate their function. A person's prescribed role may be that of the mother but she may be functioning more like a child. One's functional role can be identified by how one acts in the context of the family. Ms. Brown recently got divorced and began going out nightly with friends to various bars. She wanted to take advantage of her newfound freedom and forget about her problems and responsibilities. She would often come home late after having had too much to drink. Bella, her 16-year-old daughter, would call her mother when she was out to make sure that she was OK and take care of her when she came home. Ms. Brown was functioning more like a child and Bella like the parent. It is common, as in the Browns' case, for one family member's role to develop in response to another's. These can often operate as polarities. One child may function in the role of a family angel in response to another child being the identified patient or the one typically getting into trouble.

Flexibility and Connectedness

The assessment of subsystems, hierarchy, and boundaries provides an understanding of a family's structure, or its basic shape. The assessment of a family's flexibility and connectedness captures its *process*. By process, we mean its interactional style and emotional climate. Two interrelated processes that are part of your systemic assessment are flexibility and connectedness.

Flexibility refers to the family's ability to adapt to change, which is intimately related to the family's leadership and organization. Flexibility has two primary ingredients. First, how does the family mold and reshape its structure to accommodate change? Some families will make the necessary adjustments in roles, responsibilities, and expectations to cope effectively with change; others will resist such change. For example, a father is diagnosed with a debilitating chronic illness and is unable to perform the functions normally expected of him. His spouse and children must find ways to acknowledge and communicate about the changes associated with the illness. If the family fails to restructure their roles and responsibilities and acts as if nothing has changed, it's highly likely that stress will increase and the family's functioning will suffer. You can see similar dynamics in families coping with life cycle transitions: How will a family cope with their child transitioning to adolescence and her effort to gain more autonomy? Will the rules and expectations they had for her when she was 10 years old remain the same, or will they change to accommodate her emerging desires and needs?

A second ingredient of flexibility is continuity: How is stability maintained in the face of change? When a family is in the midst of change, they need to preserve some continuity in ways such as daily routines and rituals. For example, divorce is filled with many stressful changes for parents and children, and research has shown that too much stressful change is harmful for children (Clarke-Stewart, 2006; Terling-Watt, 2001). Children need parents who can minimize the disruptions associated with divorce and restore some semblance of predictability through rules, roles, and patterns of interaction.

Achieving flexibility means striking a delicate balance between continuity and change. The spousal subsystem helps set the tone for how this balance is achieved. Without strong, clear leadership from parents, families are susceptible to either overly rigid responses to change (too much structure and control) or overly permissive (too little structure and control), which can lead to chaos (Walsh, 2006).

While flexibility relates to control in families, connectedness relates to support in families—what is the amount of caring, closeness, and affection in the family (Olson & Gorall, 2003)? Family members need to feel secure and safe in their environment, particularly when adversity and stress are high. During times of crisis, family members are ideally turning toward one another to listen and share concerns and offer any assistance that facilitates healing and recovery. When cohesion is absent, family members feel disconnected and alone and are forced to look outside the family for needed support. In therapy, these families are hard to engage in treatment, appear to show a lack of concern or worry about serious problems, and are very disorganized, which is demonstrated in their lack of follow-through, such as completing tasks outside of therapy.

Although connectedness is usually a strength in families, too much connection can block family members' efforts to express individual differences and threatens physical and emotional privacy. When children are young, they require this high level of closeness and protection. As children move through adolescence and seek greater intellectual and behavioral freedom, too much connectedness and overprotection can feel stifling and lead to intense conflict. In therapy, these families will be easy to engage in treatment but suspicious of the input of outsiders. When questions are directed at one person, others will interject and answer for the family member. In addition, you may see an overreaction to minor problems that well-functioning families easily resolve.

As we briefly mentioned earlier and discuss at greater length in the next chapter, flexibility and connectedness are intimately related to a family's development. A family's flexibility and connectedness ideally change through the life cycle to accommodate individual development and family transitions. Families experience unpredictable transitions that can create chaos or rigidity and push a family toward more togetherness or separateness. For example, a grandparent moving into the family home may disrupt or exacerbate particular patterns. The ability of a family to work together and accommodate these changes is central to their functioning as a family.

Optimum levels of flexibility and connectedness can look different from culture to culture. In some cultures, families may function just fine with very high levels of connectedness. For example, in many Asian families, the priorities and needs of the family often supersede those of the individual. It's always important to understand family dynamics in the context of the family's culture.

The Circumplex Model: Placing Families on a Conceptual Map

The circumplex model of marital and family systems (Olson, Russell, & Sprenkle, 1989) is a useful model for integrating the concepts of family flexibility and connectedness. As you can see in Figure 9.1, flexibility ranges from rigid to chaotic. Cohesion, or connectedness, ranges from disengaged to enmeshed. Communication is a third dimension that captures how families work out issues related to cohesion and flex-

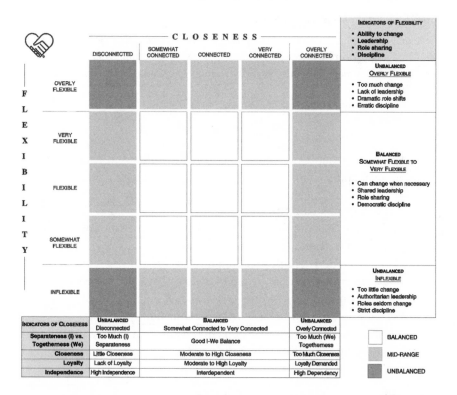

FIGURE 9.1. Circumplex model. From Olson and Gorall (2003). Copyright 2003 by The Guilford Press. Reprinted by permission.

ibility. The model allows you to place families on a conceptual map. For example, a family may have a low level of cohesion and too much flexibility (chaotically disengaged), which may be related to poor parental leadership, children who demonstrate out-of-control behavior, and communication that is unclear. The hypothesis of the model is that balanced levels of cohesion and flexibility are most conducive to healthy family functioning.

Olson, Gorall, and Tiesel (2007) developed an instrument based on the circumplex model, FACES IV, to provide a comprehensive self-report assessment of family flexibility and cohesion. Although your clinical interview and observation of family process will be the primary way you assess a family, assessment techniques like FACES IV and additional instruments listed in Table 9.1 are a helpful supplement to better understanding family dynamics.

TABLE 9.1. Family Assessment Instruments

- Family Adaptability and Cohesion Scales (FACES; Olson, Gorall, & Tiesel, 2007)
- Family Assessment Device (FAD; Epstein, Baldwin, & Bishop, 1983)
- Family Assessment Measure (FAM III; Skinner, Steinhauer, & Santa-Barbera, 1984)
- Family Environment Scale (FES; Moos & Moos, 1986)

Below are sample questions to assess flexibility and cohesiveness, which are adapted from FACES IV:

"How do you spend time together as a family?"

"When you have problem, who in the family do you talk to? How do they respond to you and the problem?"

"How often do friends and extended family visit your home?"

"How do family members respond when there is a change in plans or routines?"

"What are some of the basic rules in your family?"

"Who makes the major decisions in the family? How are these decisions communicated to the family?"

ASSESSING DIVERSE FAMILY STRUCTURES

Immigrant Families

The concepts of continuity and change are especially relevant for immigrant families—how do immigrant families continue connections with their family, culture, and nation of origin and at the same time develop new lives in their adopted country? Falicov (2007) describes the relational stress associated with separations and reunions between parents and children. It is becoming more common for Latin American mothers to leave their children in the care of relatives in order to search for work in the United States. The separations can last for many years, which creates "boundary ambiguity," or confusion about who is and isn't a part of the family (Falicov, 2002; Boss, 1998). If a reunification occurs, the initial joy and celebration is gradually replaced by children's expression of anger and resentment toward their mother for leaving home and missing years of their lives. When immigrant families arrive in therapy, you will benefit from assessing their immigration experience, particularly how presenting symptoms relate to painful separations and reunions.

Another potential challenge that immigrant families can face is conflict over the differences in acculturation between family generations. Parents who have emigrated from another country are more likely to closely follow the traditions of their country of origin. In contrast, children of immigrant families who are raised primarily in the United States may become more acculturated to American culture. These differences in cultural values can create tension or conflict between the parents and children.

Single-Parent Families

Whether the result of divorce, death, or a choice to parent alone, single-parent families, usually headed by the mother (Simmons & O'Neill, 2001), share many common challenges that have the potential to go unrecognized in the therapy room. When a child from a single-parent family is presented to you for therapy, you will benefit by identifying these challenges, most notably the possible challenges of financial stress and the fact that many single-parent families are coping with loss, whether it be the loss of a partner or parent or the loss of a dream about a family's future (Anderson, 2003).

Due to work and family demands, single parents frequently feel overwhelmed and depleted by their varied roles and responsibilities. In addition, children of single parents may carry a greater share of the domestic responsibilities because their sole parent is working outside the home. Because strands of American culture have often been critical of single-family structure, it is common for single parents to live with the guilt of "not being good enough."

While single-parent families often face daunting challenges, most of them are competent and successful. Lindblad-Goldberg (1989) has identified successful single-parent families as those in which parents, usually mothers, showed less depression, experienced more control over their lives, displayed more effective executive authority with their children, launched their older children from the household, communicated more effectively, developed close family ties, cognitively highlighted positive life experiences rather than negative ones, and utilized social networks creatively. When working with single parents or children of single parents, it is imperative that you assess their hardships as well as their strengths and resilience.

When working with single-parent families, it's important to assess what Becker and Liddle (2001) call the "self of the parent." Assessing the self of the parent means asking about hardships, such as exhaustion and work stress, as well as their efforts to care for their individual needs. Beginning therapists are frequently hesitant to do this assessment because they want to focus on the presenting problem and feel blocked by the single parent's reluctance to self-disclose. If you want to understand the interaction between single parents and their children and build a therapeutic alliance, you will need to learn more about their personal concerns outside of their role as parent (Becker & Liddle, 2001).

Gay and Lesbian Families

Due to the diversity within the gay and lesbian community, it would be a mistake to draw general conclusions about gay and lesbian families. However, it is useful to understand and assess the pathways by which gay and lesbian families are created. Ariel and McPherson (2000) describe two groups of lesbian and gay families: (1) stepfamilies that are created after the divorce of a heterosexual couple when one member begins a relationship with a same-sex partner; and (2) gay and lesbian couples having children through a variety of methods, including adoption, artificial insemination, and surrogacy. These methods usher in many family issues, such as the identification, inclusion, and rights of biological parents. Stepfamilies with gay and lesbian parents face many of same issues as any stepfamily, which are described in the next section. However, you will want to be aware of possible homophobia within the stepfamily and outside the family in the community. Ariel and McPherson (2000) offer many helpful questions for assessment of gay and lesbian stepfamilies, which include questions about the level of support of the heterosexual former spouse, the reaction of children (especially older children) to the gay or lesbian stepparent, and the reaction and level of support of extended family.

Stepfamilies

Although it's rare for a client to label a problem as a "stepfamily problem," stepfamily dynamics are a common, important undercurrent that you need to explore. In order to appropriately assess stepfamilies, you need a basic understanding of issues many stepfamilies face. We will summarize some of the key issues for stepfamily assessment. Of particular importance are the qualities of the couple's relationship, step-parent–stepchild relationships, and, in the case of divorce, the level of cooperation between former spouses in their roles as co-parents. We describe these and other issues below.

Who Is "in the Family"?

We highlighted this earlier as an important question for all families, but it's especially important for stepfamilies. You might assume that family membership is easy to define. In fact, family members in stepfamilies frequently have different definitions of who is "in" and "out" of the family. In others words, the boundaries are ambiguous. The differing definitions are due to acceptance (or a lack of acceptance) of new members and their roles in the family. For example, Stephanie, a single mother of three boys (Terrance, age 12, Vincent, 9, and Jacob, 5), remarries 6 years after their death of her husband, the father of her children. Terrance is angry with his mother for inviting a new person, especially a male, into their family home and is resentful toward this man for trying to replace his father, even though that's not the new husband's intention. Jacob is very fond of Tom, his new stepfather, and likes having a new playmate in the home. In this example, Terrance will treat his stepfather as an uninvited outsider, while Jacob will warmly welcome him as a new family member. Terrance's anger and resentment likely stem from his powerful status while his mother was a single parent, as well as his continued loyalty to his deceased father. Power issues and loyalty conflicts are common in stepfamilies and are a roadblock in a stepfamily's efforts at forming a family identity.

How Did This Family Become a Stepfamily?

An assessment of how a family became a stepfamily will inform your understanding of current issues. How much time elapsed between the end of the previous marriage or relationship and the beginning of the new couple relationship? If the new couple's relationship began prior to the ending of the previous relationship, how did the couple know each other (e.g., friends, coworkers, extramarital affair)? How was the new partner introduced to the family? When the new couple decided to marry, how were the children told? How did the family prepare for the transition to stepfamily life (e.g., roles, responsibilities, expectations)?

How Is the Couple Attending to the Needs of Their New Relationship?

Newly married (or committed) couples must find ways to protect their developing relationship; this is particularly vital for new couples in stepfamilies (Visher & Visher, 1988). Newly married couples in stepfamilies are not only coping with the adjustments associated with early marriage, such as developing problem-solving skills, but also the stress of new stepparent–stepchild relationships. Couples without children have the luxury of time to prepare their relationship for children; stepfamilies are thrust into these parent–child roles immediately, which may leave little time to nurture the new couple relationship. According to Hetherington & Stanley-Hagan (2002), marriages and children in stepfamilies fare better when spouses focus on establishing a supportive, positive marriage. Couples can be tested when conflict arises between stepparents and stepchildren and biological parents are pulled into the conflict—does the biological parent show loyalty to the child or the new spouse, or remain neutral? How do the new spousal subsystem and established biological parent–child subsystem cope with this stress?

What Developmental Stage Is the Stepfamily in?

Papernow (1993) described seven stages that stepfamilies go through:

1. Fantasy—adults have expectations of instant love in a ready-made family.
2. Immersion—a sense of discomfort and evidence of tension and conflict.
3. Awareness—members getting to know themselves and each other in the new system.
4. Mobilization—coping with struggles over differences while maintaining momentum from earlier stages.
5. Action—strengthening of the couple's relationship and greater cohesion among new family members.
6. Contact—stepparent–stepchild relationship becomes closer and more authentic and some stability has been achieved.
7. Resolution—members experience their step relationships as reliable and nurturing.

It can take stepfamilies many years to work through these stages. You may find that a family is progressing normally through the stages, which will allow you to normalize their challenges, or you may find that the family is stuck in one stage and needs help progressing to the next stage.

What Are the Agreements (and Disagreements) about Parenting the Children?

Family loyalties and role ambiguity are complicating factors in decisions about parenting responsibilities. Divorced biological parents must work out parenting issues while living in separate households, and new stepparents must work on developing a relationship with stepchildren and determining their parental role. The research suggests that children tend to reject stepparents who discipline and try to control them early on (Ganong, Coleman, Fine, & Martin, 1999). Like many new parents, couples in stepfamilies may have had very little discussion about parenting roles and methods and rely on assumed or stereotyped roles without considering the effects on the children. For example, a biological mother may hand over disciplinary responsibilities of her two boys to their new stepfather because "men are the disciplinarians," even though the children may rebel against this arrangement. Spousal disagreements about parenting practices may also be the first crisis in a new stepfamily, which isn't surprising due to the efforts to merge multiple family belief systems.

CASE EXAMPLE OF JEREMY

Jeremy, a 15-year-old boy, was referred to an outpatient community mental health center by his school due to physical altercations with peers and general anger management issues. On the phone, Jeremy's mother, Anna, a Caucasian woman in her early 30s, requested that he be seen alone to "get his anger out." The family therapist asked for the entire family to attend the first meeting, which included Jeremy, his mother, his stepfather, Roberto, a Latino man in his mid-30s, and Jeremy's 2-year-old half sister, Claudia. During the first meeting, Roberto dominated the session: He explained that Jeremy disrespected everyone in the house, especially his mother. He didn't listen to anyone or complete any of the chores required of him.

Roberto said he had taken away everything that was important to Jeremy, including his freedom after school and on weekends, but nothing had worked. As Roberto expressed his frustration, Anna was tearful and Jeremy bit at his fingernails. When the therapist asked Anna for her perspective, she says she's scared and frustrated with Jeremy. To make matters worse, she said, she was "constantly in the middle" of arguments between Roberto and Jeremy and "couldn't take it anymore." When the therapist turned to Jeremy, he was quiet initially and then stated that Roberto was not his father and couldn't tell him what to do.

The therapist's exploration of the history of the problem revealed the following information: Anna said Jeremy changed significantly after she and Roberto met and moved in together. Anna and Jeremy moved in with Roberto in early March 2006, 1 week after Anna and Roberto first met. Prior to moving in with Roberto, Anna and Jeremy lived with Anna's mother, who died in late January 2006 after a long illness. Jeremy stated that he was very close to his grandmother; she was like a "second mom" to him. Prior to moving in with Roberto, there was no discussion between Anna, Jeremy, and Roberto about parenting roles and responsibilities. Roberto stated that he assumed he would be the disciplinarian because he was "the man of the house" and Jeremy didn't have a father (note: Jeremy never met his father).

Therapist's Presession and First-Session Observations

- The school referred Jeremy.
- Mom initially requested individual therapy.
- The whole family arrived for the first session, as requested.
- Roberto dominated the session. He appeared to care for his new family.
- Mom was very passive and appeared depressed.
- Jeremy was very quiet and appeared angry.
- Claudia was playful and appeared happy.
- Anna and Jeremy have experienced significant losses: Anna's mother (Jeremy's grandmother), loss of home, loss of neighborhood, loss of school, loss of friends.
- Anna, Jeremy, and Roberto had very little preparation in their transition to becoming a stepfamily. The stepfamily never discussed roles and responsibilities of each family member.

Therapist's Notes about the Family's Structure and Process

- The family has diffuse internal and external boundaries, as evident by the ease with which Roberto stepped into a disciplinary role with Jeremy.
- There is an unhealthy hierarchy in the spousal subsystem—Roberto appears to possess more power than Anna. At times, Anna seems like Jeremy's sibling, which is another example of their diffuse internal boundaries.
- There is a central triangle between Roberto, Anna, and Jeremy.
- The family is engaged in the following interactional pattern (Figure 9.2): Jeremy misbehaves at home, mother tells stepfather about misbehavior, stepfather gets angry and punishes Jeremy, mother is silent; Jeremy feels hurt, angry, and abandoned by his mother's silence, Jeremy acts out because he is hurt by his mother's inaction.
- The family demonstrates a high level of flexibility, bordering on chaotic.
- The family demonstrates a moderate level of connectedness, at times moving toward disengagement.
- The roles and responsibilities of each family member have been implicit, rather than explicit, particularly Roberto's role as stepfather.
- Roberto's strong involvement may have something to do with his wanting to be seen as the head of the household, which may be related to both gender and cultural expectations.

The therapist would take this preliminary data and merge it with other assessment information, including details about Roberto's and Anna's families of origin, their own development as a family, and their relationship with the community, all of which will be discussed in the next chapter.

INTEGRATING FAMILY FUNCTIONING AND INDIVIDUAL FUNCTIONING

Since family and individual functioning can exert a bidirectional influence on each other, family therapists must maintain simultaneous awareness of both. Family therapists strongly believe family func-

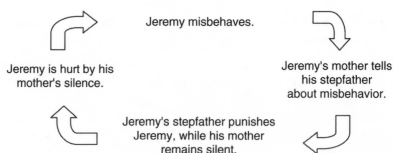

FIGURE 9.2. Interactional cycle for Jeremy's family.

tioning has a powerful influence on child and adolescent well-being. Children triangulated in parental conflict may act out or develop some form of psychopathology such as depression. Improper hierarchies or boundaries can also lead to problems in terms of child and adolescent functioning.

However, individual functioning can also impact family functioning. Adult psychopathology or well-being, for example, can impact family dynamics. A parent with ADHD may have a difficult time providing his or her child with ADHD with the necessary structured environment. Or, a father may become disengaged with his children due to his chronic depression.

A child's or adolescent's psychopathology may also impact family dynamics. Parents may become preoccupied with managing one child's psychopathology, which detracts them from attending to the needs of their other children. Thus, a triangle can be created where the parents become enmeshed with the child suffering from mental illness, and become disengaged from the other children. Due to jealousy, the siblings may resent the child who is getting a disproportionate share of the parents' attention. Parents may also disagree on how to handle the child's psychopathology, which may create parental or couple discord. Therefore, as family therapists, we must be comfortable shifting back and forth between assessing individual and family functioning.

CONCLUSION

Regardless of whether your client is an individual, couple, or family, a comprehensive, systemic family assessment is essential and serves as a foundation for your work as a family therapist. While one might assume that all family therapists routinely do family assessments, we have been surprised at how seldom families are considered in assessment, particularly when an individual is the presenting client. For example, our students will sometimes treat seriously ill adult parents, often single parents, and fail to inquire about the welfare of their dependent children. Family assessment takes time, is more complicated, and can be overwhelming for new therapists attempting to make sense of a large amount of clinical data. However, good family assessments are worth the time and will provide you with an invaluable picture of the interactional patterns that contribute to your client's presenting problems.

CHAPTER 10

Assessing the Multigenerational Family through Time

In the previous chapter, we discussed assessment of family interaction in the here and now. However, in order to fully understand how family members interact, it's essential to learn about the relevant contexts for their behavior. For example, the case example at the end of Chapter 9 included a stepfather, Roberto, who was struggling with how to develop a relationship with and discipline his stepson, Jeremy. Through an exploration of the Roberto's family of origin, the therapist learned that Roberto's father had used harsh, physically abusive methods of discipline with him. Roberto said he "escaped" his home when he turned 18, frequently living on the street due to his lack of money. After Jeremy's birth, his mother, Anna, moved in and out of her mother's home, leaving Jeremy with her mother and never fully assuming the role of primary parent. After the death of her mother, Anna and Jeremy immediately moved in with Roberto and, again, Anna never fully assumed a leadership role as a parent. The family-of-origin information helped the therapist understand the context of their current family structure.

When clients arrive for therapy, they are commonly overwhelmed and immobilized by their current challenges, a fact that tends to magnify the present moment and deemphasize contextual variables that could be contributing to their stress (McGoldrick & Carter, 2003;

Nichols & Everett, 1986). Like their clients, therapists can also become overly focused on the current crisis rather than broadening their perspective to understand the larger picture. A multigenerational, developmental perspective is valuable in two primary ways: First, it allows you to explore and understand dysfunctional patterns throughout the system over time, not just in the present moment; and second, it helps you identify predictable and unpredictable changes in a system's natural growth and development. Predictable changes include the movement between life cycle stages, such as the transition to adolescence. Unpredictable changes could include job loss, geographical relocation and migration, serious illness, divorce, or other events that have a major impact on family life.

The ability of a family to work together and accommodate developmental changes is central to its functioning as a family. According to Nichols and Everett (1986), "Some families may present themselves for therapy at the onset of the [developmental] disruption, others may not feel that there is a problem until disruptive events have accumulated and ... resulted in severe symptomatology" (p. 186). The family therapist hypothesizes that the presenting problem may have a lot to do with the family being stuck in its progress toward achieving a particular developmental stage. For example, the 14-year-old daughter of very controlling parents may start "acting out" by breaking curfew and hanging out at school with people the parents deem unacceptable. This behavior signals a difficulty in the family system's transition to the "family with adolescents" stage, where there is a need to increase the permeability of the family boundary to include the teenager's growing independence.

In this chapter, we will focus on assessing the "big picture," including the multigenerational family, the family's movement over time, and the family's interaction with the community. Taking a multigenerational, historical perspective doesn't mean looking for a cause in the past to explain the present. Rather, our emphasis is on exploring the continuation of patterns, emotions, and behaviors over at least three generations and understanding the changes that have taken place in a family over the recent and distant past. Three related assessment maps will be discussed below: (1) genograms, (2) timelines, and (3) sociograms. All three maps work in concert with one another to better understand your client. We use the following case example to illustrate each map:

Bob and Gabriela Barber arrive for counseling presenting both marital and family problems. Bob, age 53, is Caucasian and was born and raised in the United States. Gabriela, age 51, was born in Brazil and came to the United States when she was in her mid-20s. They have been married for 23 years. Their current concern is their 21-year-old daughter, Tania, who recently quit college after her fiancé broke off their engagement. She recently returned home to live with her parents. Tania has been staying out late at night, going to bars and parties with friends. She sleeps until late in the morning and fails to do what is asked of her around the house. She says that she will eventually get a part-time job, but for now she says she just needs some time to figure things out. Bob and Gabriela disagree about how to handle this situation. Bob thinks that they should adopt a "tough love policy" and set rules for Tania. He believes that they should not give her any money and should take away her car until she gets a job. Gabriela believes that Tania is confused and needs time. She would like to avoid putting any pressure on Tania and give her a chance to sort her life out. The family difficulties are complicated further by the recent arrival of Gabriela's 82-year-old mother, who moved to the United States from Brazil 1 year ago following the death of her husband from Alzheimer's disease. He was a workaholic and left Gabriela's mother in a very financially secure position. Gabriela didn't want her mother to live alone and thought it would be best for her to live with them. Gabriela's mother has several physical ailments, including arthritis and chronic pain, and is receiving treatment that she frustratingly says isn't effective. She believes that Bob is too strict with Tania and she secretly gives Gabriela money on a regular basis.

Tania has a younger brother, Felipe, who is in his first year of college. He has had little contact with the family since he went off to school. The parents are concerned about his drug use, which started in middle school. Due to the recession in 2009, the tuition support provided by his public university has been cut, which has added to the financial stress in the family. Bob and Gabriela argue constantly about how to handle the problems with Tania and with Gabriela's mother. They are both frustrated and think the situation is out of control. Bob blames Gabriela for inviting her mother to stay with them for so long. He thought that she would only be there for a month or two and it has turned into a year. Bob is particularly upset about feeling "ganged up on" by Gabriela and her mother. He says that sometimes they both yell and curse at him in Portuguese. He has threatened to leave the home if his mother-in-law stays much longer. Bob is also feeling extreme financial stress due to layoffs at his business. He is a district sales manager and the sales in his region have been very low, which has him worried that he might lose his job. Gabriela worked part time as sales representative until she lost her job 3 months ago. She feels strongly that it is important to take care of her family and help them as much as she can. She is overwhelmed by the stress of the problems with her family and has been suffering from depression and back pain. She was originally treated for depression 10 years ago when she suspected that her husband was having an affair. She is still not sure if this occurred. Bob began receiving treatment for alcohol abuse at about this same time. He has continued attending weekly Alcoholics Anonymous meetings and claims to have been sober for the last 7 years. Gabriela is currently being treated with antidepressant medication. She also has a history of taking medication for pain.

GENOGRAMS: ASSESSING THE MULTIGENERATIONAL FAMILY

A genogram is used for a variety of purposes in therapy. In some cases, it takes on a very minor role, such as helping to organize a therapist's private notes that may or may not include family-of-origin data. For example, during a first session a therapist might draw a genogram in her notes to keep track of who is in the family. In other cases, the genogram takes on a starring role and becomes a focus of treatment, which is a common method in the transgenerational approaches to family therapy (Kerr & Bowen, 1988). We see the genogram as much more than a note-taking tool, but not a sole treatment technique. The construction of a genogram with the family is an essential part of any comprehensive assessment, helping us appreciate the family's current challenges and strengths. We have seen many students skip this part of the assessment and regret it later when they're stuck, or when important family-of-origin information arises later in treatment and they feel foolish for not knowing the information.

Genogram Basics

In its simplest form, a genogram is a visual map to identify members of a family, including gender, generation, and age. Figure 10.1 provides a

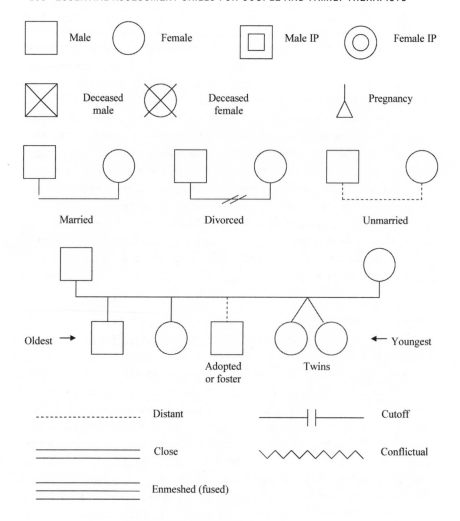

FIGURE 10.1. Common genogram symbols.

summary of the most commonly used symbols for the graphic depiction of a family (McGoldrick, Gerson, & Petry, 2008; Pendegast & Sherman, 1977). We won't describe each symbol, but rather highlight a few of the most relevant symbols. Each family member is represented by a square (male) or a circle (female); ages are written in each symbol. The identified client or patient (IP) is indicated with concentric squares or circles. Siblings are listed based in their birth order, oldest to youngest from left to right. The youngest generation is drawn at the bottom, with the oldest generations above the younger generations. Marriages are indicated with a solid line; the husband goes on the left. Committed relationships are indicated with a dotted line. Previous or subsequent marital or committed relationships are drawn on the left or right side. At times, you will want to record information that either doesn't have a symbol or has one you can't remember. In situations like this, give yourself permission to improvise by writing statements on the genogram or creating your own symbols. The genogram does not need to look perfect; it just needs to communicate the important information.

The Construction of a Genogram

Early in your work with a client, preferably in the second session, you will be setting aside time to collect information for a three- or four-generation genogram. By this time, most therapists have already been constructing a genogram in their private notes in order to organize all the information they've received. Including family members in a discussion about extended family changes the genogram from a note-taking tool to an assessment tool. Because your client will be focused on the presenting problem, questions may be raised about why precious time is being used to gather information "in the past." You need to be prepared to present a rationale for why the information is important (e.g., "What we learned in our families growing up often influences our attitudes and behaviors in our current relationships"; "I want to know about the strengths and resources in your family that will help you overcome this problem"). If you don't view the information as important, it will be very difficult to convince your client that it's important. Most clients will understand the importance of doing "a good history" because it's consistent with their experiences seeing other health care professionals.

　　Once you and your client agree to do a genogram, your next challenge is how to stay on task. Some therapists prepare for these interviews and then get sidetracked when clients present a flurry of new issues since the previous session. Although you need to give priority to crises, such as suicide ideation or abuse, most new issues can wait to be addressed until after a thorough assessment. In order to help your clients stay focused, we recommend constructing the genogram on a large piece of paper that everyone can clearly see. You can keep the genogram in your file and post it on the wall during each session. Another advantage of a large poster is that you can involve children in the drawing of symbols and lines, which engages them in therapy and may provide diagnostic information based on how they diagram particular relationships.

The first phase in the construction of a genogram is breadth. Here is a list of the information we gather first:

- Gender, age, and name of each family member, starting with the youngest and moving up.[1]
- For family members who have died, list the person's age at the time of death, along with an X inside their symbol to indicate the loss. Also, indicate how the person died.[2]
- Connect the family members with lines indicating biological or legal relationships.
- On the relationship lines, make a note of the beginning and, if needed, ending dates of relationships.

The second phase in the construction of a genogram is depth. Here is a list of the information we gather:

- Descriptions of each relevant family member. "Let's start with your father. Tell me a little bit about him." For clients who need more structure, you may want to ask the following: "What are five words that describe your father?" Regardless of how you gather the information, you will want to make sure that positive descriptions are included with negative descriptions.
- A description of how your client believes other family members would describe him or her. "If your parents and siblings were here, how would they describe you?" or "What are five words your parents and siblings would use to describe you?" These descriptions can frequently capture roles in a family (e.g., scapegoat, star, black sheep, comedian).
- Descriptions of dyadic relationships. "Tell me about the rela-

---

[1] A common question is whether you need to include every distant relative. Although in some cases it might be necessary to get this specific, we recommend focusing on the closest family members.

[2] Unless it's relevant to the presenting problem, avoid spending too much time at this stage on the circumstances of a death. You can acknowledge the significance of a loss and ask the family if you can revisit the experience at a later date.

tionship between you and your father? What about the relationship between you and your sister? What about the relationship between your parents? How have these relationships changed over time?"

- Description of family time together. "What was a typical day in the life of your family? What did your family do for fun together?"
- Description of the family emotional climate. "How were anger, sadness, and joy expressed in your family? If you had a problem, who did you go talk to? If your parents were unhappy with your behavior, how did they discipline you?" These descriptions can capture rules in a family—both explicit (e.g., "no dating until you're 16") and implicit (e.g., "we don't talk about a family member after they've died").
- Family belief systems and mantras. "What were some of the core beliefs in your family?" For example, families may carry beliefs related to gender (e.g., men should not be vulnerable or show emotions other than anger) and what is normal or abnormal ("We have a great relationship; we never argue") (Rolland, 1994).

Figure 10.2 provides an illustration of the Barber family after both phases.

By this point, you will have heard many descriptions of family members and relationships, and general themes will begin to emerge, that may or may not connect to the presenting problem. Themes are often identified as patterns in the family's functioning that occur across generations. In the Barber family, there are four prominent patterns: (1) a pattern of substance abuse (Gabriela's father, Bob, Gabriela, and Felipe—crosses three generations); (2) a pattern of secrets, including alleged affairs and questions about money; (3) a pattern of gender roles (men provide financial support and security, women are the primary caretakers and align with children); and (4) a pattern of unresolved conflict in spousal and parent–child subsystems. Other examples of positive and negative patterns in families include depression, emotional instability, cutting off family members, resilience in coping with stress, bonding together in the face of loss, abandonment, and physical or verbal abuse. Although a genogram can become a focus of treatment, we're recommending the completion of a genogram during assessment

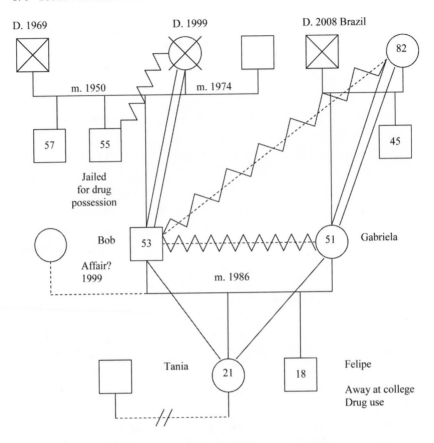

FIGURE 10.2. Genogram of the Barber family.

in order to rule in and rule out specific issues, such as transgenerational patterns, as you and your client decide on treatment goals.

Although a genogram is a valuable tool for identifying the "vertical" stressors (e.g., relationship patterns, addictions, violence) in the life a family (McGoldrick & Carter, 2003), it obscures the temporal dimension of family history (Friedman, Rohrbaugh, & Krakauer, 1988). In other words, the genogram lists dates and events, but doesn't arrange them so their proper order can be appreciated. For example, a divorce, a move, and the diagnosis of a parent's illness may have occurred in close time proximity, which may have also been the time when a presenting problem started. We now turn our attention to the second map for multigenerational family assessment: the timeline.

TIMELINES: ASSESSMENT OF
FAMILY TRANSITIONS

A timeline works in collaboration with a genogram to note the key events in the life of a family, which can include predictable life cycle transitions, such as marriages, births, and deaths, as well as shifts and traumas in the family, such as migrations, job changes, illnesses, and divorces. Of the many benefits the timeline (Stanton, 1992; Weber & Levine, 1995) provides in family assessment, we want to highlight three primary ones:

1. It helps answer the questions "Why is the family seeking help at this particular time?" and "Is the presenting problem associated with normal aspects of a family's current stage of development or is it associated with a current or recent transition?"
2. It helps you, the therapist, understand how the family coped with other developmental challenges, which may allow you to harness a family's strengths to cope with the current challenges.
3. It adds significance to events previously considered unimportant or unappreciated in the life of the family.

It is very rare for a family to arrive in therapy and state directly that their presenting problem is a stressful transition. Your role as a professional is to connect the dots that up until now have gone unacknowledged.

As with the construction of the genogram, you will want to post a sheet of paper on the wall and allow the clients to identify the most important events, along with dates, in the life of their family. Stanton (1992) succinctly and clearly describes the process:

> It consists of drawing a long horizontal line and dividing it into equal time segments representing years, months, weeks, even days, depending on the therapist's preference. At points along the line various nodal or life cycle events are designated by short vertical markers extending downward from identifying inscriptions (e.g., "Louise loses job," "Bert and Marie get married," "William dies"). There is no limit to the kinds of nodal events that can be highlighted. They usually include key births, deaths, engagements, marriages, separations, divorces, school changes, launchings, layoffs, promotions, financial setbacks, relocations, immigrations, and the onset of severe medical events such as illnesses, hospitalizations, and surgery. Any kind of loss, gain, or change is grist for the mill (p. 332).

Figure 10.3 illustrates the Barber family's timeline. Once events are plotted on the timeline, you can begin to hypothesize the significance of particular transitions. The Barber family has recently experienced multiple significant stressful transitions, most notably around the arrival (Tania, Gabriele's mother) and departure (Felipe) of key family members, which has increased anxiety, brought forward new issues (e.g., financial stress), and reawakened unresolved issues from earlier transitions (e.g., depression, marital conflict, loss). Below, we describe some of the key predictable and unpredictable transitions that families like the Barbers face over time. First, we want to briefly summarize relevant conceptual models of family development.

Conceptualizing Families through Time

Many developmental theories and models have informed the work of family therapists (Nichols & Pace-Nichols, 2000). Carter and McGoldrick's (2005) family life cycle is the model most familiar to family therapists. It identifies tasks for families in each developmental stage and hypothesizes that stress is often greatest at transition points from one stage to another. The traditional family life cycle has received much criticism, mostly due to its assumption of universality—not all families will have children and there is no "right" way to transition from one stage to the next. Each family will be guided by its intergenerational history and the belief systems of its race, culture, and ethnicity. Even though there's tremendous variation, most families share a common process of development that includes a wide variety of stressful transitions.

Combrinck-Graham's (1985) family life spiral describes a process of family development. She states that families naturally oscillate through times of greater closeness (centripetal periods), such as the birth of a new baby, and times of greater distance (centrifugal periods), such as a child leaving home following adolescence. Centripetal periods are characterized by greater family cohesion and greater focus on internal family life. Centrifugal periods display an opening of external family boundaries, allowing individual family members to pursue goals and interactions within the extrafamilial environment. A crisis in the family, such as the onset of physical illness, generally has a centripetal pull on families. If a crisis emerges during a transition from a centripetal period to a centrifugal period (e.g., the launching of children), it may prolong the centripetal period (e.g., keeping the launching child at home longer and changing plans for college and/or career). These theories and models

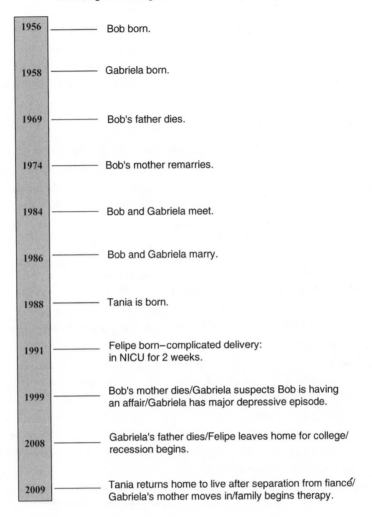

1956	———	Bob born.
1958	———	Gabriela born.
1969	———	Bob's father dies.
1974	———	Bob's mother remarries.
1984	———	Bob and Gabriela meet.
1986	———	Bob and Gabriela marry.
1988	———	Tania is born.
1991	———	Felipe born–complicated delivery: in NICU for 2 weeks.
1999	———	Bob's mother dies/Gabriela suspects Bob is having an affair/Gabriela has major depressive episode.
2008	———	Gabriela's father dies/Felipe leaves home for college/ recession begins.
2009	———	Tania returns home to live after separation from fiancé/ Gabriela's mother moves in/family begins therapy.

FIGURE 10.3. Timeline of the Barber family.

will help guide your assessment of families over time, as you encounter common themes of the traditional life cycle transitions described below and family traumas such as illness and death, all of which may be intimately connected to the problems presented by your clients.

Common Family Life Cycle Transitions

Here is a brief review of three common family life cycle transitions: (1) the transition to marriage; (2) the transition to parenthood; and (3) co-occurring transitions: launching children and later life. We recognize that there are many more life cycle stages. We are choosing to highlight the assessment of these three stages with the understanding that you have access to many resources that explore the traditional family life cycle.

The Transition to Marriage

Along with the joys of long-term commitment comes the stress of adapting to a new set of expectations and responsibilities—living space may now be shared, finances are likely integrated, new relationships with in-laws are being negotiated. Couples new to marriage may carry the assumption that marriage will usher in many new positive changes, which is true. Newly married couples experience the joys and comfort of a long-term commitment that strengthens their mutual support and ushers in many new caring behaviors. Something that doesn't appear to change when a couple marries is their conflict—there appears to be little change in levels of conflict after marriage and destructive ways of dealing with conflict remain stable or increase slightly (Noller, Feeney, Bonnell, & Callan, 1994).

In addition to communication and conflict resolution skills, which are discussed in more detail in Chapter 11, an important area of assessment with newly married couples is the development of their identity as a couple: What are the boundaries between their marriage and peers, their marriage and work, and their marriage and families of origin? If a couple marries in their 20s, which is a common age for first marriages, both partners are going through multiple transitions associated with their individual development, including: (1) differentiating sufficiently from family of origin to become an autonomous person, (2) making progress toward career aspirations, and (3) continuing old friendships and establishing new social relationships. If a person is struggling in any of these areas, it can contribute to problems in the new marriage (Nichols, 1996). For example, we've seen many new couples struggle due to diffuse boundaries with friends. One partner wants to continue to spend late nights with single friends, which breeds resentment in the other partner, who expects the new marital relationship to take priority over old friendships. When these concerns are communicated, the spouse who wants to spend time with friends feels "stifled" and accuses the other of trying to be his or her parent, which introduces a myriad of family-of-origin issues.

Chapters 11 and 12 will fully address the assessment of couples. Here are a few questions that will help you better understand your clients' transition to marriage:

> "How did your families react to the news that you were getting married?"
> "What were the best and most challenging aspects of being married?"
> "How did marriage change and not change your relationship?"
> "How did your view of yourself change after getting married?"
> "How did being married meet, exceed, or fall short of your expectations?"
> "How did your relationships with your friends and families of origin change after you got married?"

Chapter 12 discusses the unique issues faced by gay and lesbian couples in their transition to long-term commitment and marriage. As you will see next, a strong couple identity with firm boundaries is the foundation for successful future family transitions.

The Transition to Parenthood

In 1957, LeMasters claimed that 83% of new parents go through a moderate to severe crisis in the transition to parenthood. At the time, such a claim was met with public consternation due to the assumption that parenthood should be a time of pure bliss, but it's now generally accepted that the transition to parenthood can be stressful for couples (Shapiro & Gottman, 2005). Although parenthood ushers in tremendous happiness for most couples, the transition to parenthood poses two major challenges: (1) the impact it has on the marriage or relationship; and (2) the challenges of learning the skills needed to be an effective parent.

Many studies have shown that after the birth of a child, marital conflict increases (Belsky & Kelly, 1994) and marital quality decreases (Shapiro, Gottman, & Carrere, 2000). Considering the sleeplessness, fatigue, and irritability associated with caring for a new baby, as well as the lack of time available for conversation and sexual activity, it's not surprising that a couple's relationship suffers in the early stages of parenthood. A key question for couples during and beyond their transition to parenthood is "What are our expectations about the division of household labor, including caring for our new baby, and how do we evaluate our current division of labor?" Much of a couple's marital conflict typically centers on the inequities of the father's versus mother's involvement in the family (Cowan & Cowan, 2000). Women can feel overburdened by role overload—in addition to caring for a baby, they are continuing to manage their preparenthood household responsibilities. Men, on the other hand, can feel excluded from the care of the baby for many reasons, such as their own or others' low expectations about their caregiving abilities. Increased marital conflict combined with feelings of incompetence in their new parenting role can cause fathers to withdraw from their families, with both short-term and long-term negative consequences for the family.

Here are questions that explore the impact of parenthood on a couple's relationship:

> "At what point in your life did you know you wanted to be a parent?"
> "When did the two of you start discussions about having a baby?"
> "How long did it take to get pregnant?"
> [If infertile] "How did you eventually become a parent (e.g., infertility treatment, adoption)? How did this experience impact your views on being a parent?"
> "What were the biggest challenges you faced during pregnancy?"
> "What was it like during the first month after having your baby?"
> "How did your relationship change once your baby arrived?"
> "How did the two of you maintain a connection during this transition?"

As children get older, the themes of relationship equity, relationship conflict, and family inclusion become paramount as couples attend to the emotional lives of their children (Gottman, DeClaire, & Siegel, 1997) and figure out methods of becoming effective parents. Here are questions that explore this advanced part of the transition:

> "What are the ingredients that make a good parent?"
> "How are your beliefs about parenting shaped by your families of origin?"
> "What did you like and dislike about how your parents parented you?"
> "How are the two of you merging your beliefs about parenting to form a coherent, consistent approach to parenting?"

Williams and Cushing (2005) described four C's of parenting: consequences, consistency, calm, and charged batteries. The first two C's, administering consequences and doing so in a consistent manner, are an integral part of most parent management programs. These concepts are rooted in the behavioral therapy tradition, where positive reinforcement and punishment are used to shape behavior. The third C, remaining calm while administering consequences, encourages parents to be nonreactive, which helps reduce the level of negativity in the parent–child relationship. Finally, the fourth C, maintaining charged batteries, recognizes that effective parenting is difficult to do if one's personal resources are depleted. Therapists can easily use the four C's as a checklist for assessing a client's potential strengths or growth areas with regards to parenting. Based on the four C's, here are four questions that we think are important in assessing parenting:

• *What consequences are used when your child misbehaves?*" If a child misbehaves by breaking a rule, for example, then the parent is expected to attach a consequence to the behavior. Ideally, the consequence or punishment will fit the crime.

• *How consistently are these consequences used?*" Attaching consequences to behavior is most effective when done consistently. If children only occasionally receive consequences for breaking a rule, then they may continue to misbehave out of the belief that they can get away with it most of the time. Being consistent also reassures children that parents can be depended upon, not only for setting limits, but also for protecting or insuring their welfare. To the extent possible, both parents (or other caretakers who are in a parenting role) should try to follow the same rules and be consistent in giving consequences. This avoids giving children mixed messages, and reduces the likelihood that they will take advantage of the parents not having a united front.

• *How do you remain calm when your child is upset?*" Remaining calm helps keep children from assuming they are being punished simply because the parent is upset rather than for breaking a rule. In other words, the children may focus more on the fact that the parent is upset or angry than the lesson to be learned from the consequence. Children who sense that they can make their parents upset may enjoy having this kind of power or influence over their parents. As result, the child may continue to act out as a way of maintaining power over the parent. Parental power comes from giving consequences, not by becoming upset.

- *How do you charge your batteries when you feel exhausted?*" Coming up with consequences, administering them in a consistent manner, and remaining calm are all very difficult if a parent's personal batteries are run down. Therefore, an important aspect of parenting is keeping one's batteries charged. Possible factors that may contribute to parents having poorly charged batteries include depression, health problems, stress, or limited resources.

Co-Occurring Transitions: Launching Children and Later Life

Issues around launching children and caring for aging family members become more prominent as life expectancy increases. Families are challenged to accept multiple comings and goings in the family system's membership. In-laws, grandchildren, returning children, aging parents, and death must be accommodated during this life stage. Adolescents grow into adults who may have their own children, and shift from parent–child to adult–adult connections. Disease, retirement, and disability challenge the family's resources at many turns. Additions and losses pervade the emotional terrain. Adults in middle age are often caught in the middle of these intense transitions, as they attempt to support their children transitioning to adulthood and care for aging parents whose health may be deteriorating, which may require altering the decision-making structure to insure the impaired older adult is safe (Qualls, 2000).

We've stressed the importance of individual assessment throughout this book. Nowhere is this more important than in the assessment of families coping with aging family members. The diagnostic information provided in Chapter 6, particularly in the areas of depression and anxiety, will assist you in assessing common individual issues in later life. Two essential areas for assessment of later-life families include physical health and the well-being of family caregivers. Although there's tremendous variability in the health of older adults—some are very healthy while others may be facing terminal illnesses—you need to have a thorough understanding of the health of your older clients from multiple perspectives, including your clients, their family members, and their health care providers (Shields, King, & Wynne, 1995). Severe cognitive impairment affects 4.9% of adults over the age of 65 and 16–30% of those over the age of 85 (Regier, Boyd, Burke, & Rae, 1988; Skoog, Nilsson, Palmertz, Andreasson, & Svanborg, 1993). Family members are typically on the front line of care for these impaired adults. A typical patient with dementia gradually experiences the loss of problem-solving skills and executive functions, such as planning and memory, which makes it increasingly difficult to participate in normal daily activities (Qualls, 2000). As family members respond to these changes by taking on more and more responsibilities, stress builds and the potential for caregiver burnout is high. It's imperative that you explore the well-being of all family members when an older adult is experiencing cognitive deterioration.

Along with their mental and physical health challenges, older adults come to therapy with long, rich histories that highlight many relevant issues, which deserve space in the your assessment. In exploring your older adult client's personal and cultural history (Shields et al., 1995), here are a few key questions that can elicit key life narratives:

"In your reflections on your life to date, what are you most proud of?"
"What personal qualities helped make these experiences successful?"
"What have been the biggest challenges you've faced?"
"How have you been impacted by these challenges?"

Unpredictable Transitions

Illness

John Rolland (1994) described a typology of illness as a framework for understanding the diverse ways families cope with a variety of physical illnesses. He identified the following variables in his typology: onset, course, outcome, and degree of incapacitation. Onset of illness refers to whether it is acute, like stroke, or gradual, like Alzheimer's disease. A family will likely respond to an acute illness differently from one with a gradual onset. For example, an acute illness will quickly mobilize the family and force them to utilize crisis-management skills. Some families will handle this rapid change better than others. The course of an illness can be progressive (type 1 diabetes), constant (spinal cord injury), or relapsing-episodic (asthma). Relapsing illnesses create tremendous unpredictability in families. Further, they demand flexibility in the family structure due to the transitions between crisis and noncrisis periods and ongoing worry about when the next crisis will take place. The illness outcome refers to a continuum that ranges from shortening one's life span to causing the likely death of a patient. Some illnesses are nonfatal, such as arthritis, whereas others, such as Huntington's disease, are fatal. Incapacitation refers to the degree of a patient's disability—incapacitating (Alzheimer's disease) or nonincapacitating (hypertension).

Another helpful aspect of Rolland's model is the interface between the illness and the family's developmental stage, which allows one to appreciate the unique and complex effects of illness on a family. According to Rolland, the onset of physical illness generally has a centripetal pull on families. An illness that emerges during a centripetal period may prolong this period or result in a family getting stuck in this phase of development. When an illness strikes during a centrifugal period, it can interrupt a family's natural developmental progression and force its members to redirect their attention back to the family. A common example is a child in late adolescence remaining at home beyond the time she originally expected in order to help care for an ill parent.

Ruddy and McDaniel (2008) and Rolland (1994) list questions for the assessment of families coping with illness. Below is a sample of their questions:

> "What do you think caused this illness?"
> "How do you think typical families cope with this kind of illness?"
> "What changes in family responsibilities do you think will be needed because of the patient's sickness?"
> "If the patient needs care or special help, what family members are going to be responsible for providing it?"
> "If the illness is already chronic or appears likely to become chronic, what are the patient's and family members' plans for taking care of the problem over the long term?"
> "What has been your extended family's experience with illness?"

Death

Of all the transitions that families experience, death might be the most profound, due to its wide and far-reaching effects (Bowen, 1991; Horwitz, 1997). Death is rarely contained in one period of time; rather, it can dramatically alter the family's anticipated life course for generations. For example, the loss of a parent during childhood is often revisited throughout one's life, during moments of celebration, such as graduations and births, and during moments of sadness, such as subsequent losses. During your assessments, we strongly recommend exploring both recent and distant losses. A recent loss may be the reason a family is coming to therapy. However, clients seldom arrive at therapy with unresolved grief as their presenting problem, and they frequently have little understanding of the possible connection between their current problems and unresolved grief. Although we're not suggesting that unresolved grief is the foundation for every presenting problem, we do believe that listening to stories of death is an essential part of family assessment.

Historically, the assessment of grief has focused on stages, phases, and tasks that *individuals* experience during grief. For example, Bowlby (1980) and Parkes (1972) describe a general grief process that starts with disorganization (e.g., emotional numbness, denial), followed by a period of extremes (e.g., searching for the deceased, accommodating the loss), and then eventually resolution or acceptance of the loss. More recently, the emphasis has shifted from stages and phases of grief to assessing an individual's complicated grief, which includes: (1) a sense of disbelief regarding the death; (2) anger and bitterness over the death; (3) recurrent pangs of painful emotions, with intense yearning and longing for the deceased; and (4) preoccupation with thoughts of the loved one, often including distressing intrusive thoughts related to the death (Horwitz et al., 1997; Shear, Frank, Houck, & Reynolds, 2005).

Besides clinical attention to emotionally distressed individuals, we want you to use your systemic perspective to appreciate the reverberation of death throughout the family network, including an assessment of the immediate and long-term impact of death for partners, parents, children, siblings, and extended family (Walsh, 2006). Here is a list of sample questions that can help you understand a family's response to death:

- What are the complicating factors associated with this loss (e.g., untimely loss, sudden death, violent death, suicide, conflict in the relationship with the deceased, perceived preventability of the death, lack of social support)?
- How did the family grieve the loss? What rituals, if any, did they use?
- How did/do they communicate with each other about the loss?
- What are the family's beliefs about why the loss occurred?

- What changed and did not change during the dying process and after the death (e.g., changes in roles and responsibilities, changes in relationship closeness)?
- How is the family balancing change with the continuity of familiar patterns?
- What concurrent transitions took place or are taking place in addition to the death (e.g., moving, life cycle transitions, job changes)?
- What have been the multiple losses created by the death (e.g., loss of the person, loss of roles and relationships, the loss of the intact family unit, loss of hopes and dreams for what might have been) (Walsh, 2006)?
- How has the family coped with previous losses? What was learned in these previous losses that might be useful in coping with recent losses?

SOCIOGRAMS: ASSESSING FAMILIES AND COMMUNITY SYSTEMS

In addition to considering the interactions within multigenerational families over time, it is vital to consider the interactions between families and social systems in the community in your assessments. Many families are engaged in meaningful, and sometimes stressful, relationships with nonfamily resources, including friends, neighbors, teachers, physicians, social workers, probation officers, and others. For example, when a family member is diagnosed with physical illness, the family is thrust into the medical community, which requires interactions with physicians, nurses, office staff, insurance companies, and many others. Families who have had bad experiences and have negative beliefs about the medical community may have a difficult time developing good working relationships with the health care team (Ruddy & McDaniel, 2008). Inquiring about community support might also uncover a dearth of supportive resources, which will inform your treatment plan.

A sociogram can be drawn to map out the larger systems currently active in a family's life. The map can be drawn in a variety of ways. Based on their work with gay and lesbian couples, Green and Mitchell (2008) draw the sociogram as five concentric circles, which are labeled as follows: the couple (the innermost circle);

very close/supportive ties; close supportive ties; instrumental ties/ acquaintances; and others (the outermost circle). To diagram the relationships between family members and community systems without creating too many separate maps, we prefer to integrate the sociogram with the genogram by drawing multiple large circles above the genogram. The systems and issues that could be drawn above the Barbers' genogram include the health care system (relationship between Gabriela's mother and her doctors), the educational system (Felipe in college), Bob's work system, and the global economic recession, which is impacting every system. As you draw the sociogram, here are a few questions to consider about the links between your clients and community systems:

- How do family members view the community systems that currently impact their lives?
- How are community systems complicating and/or improving your client's life?
- What patterns currently exist in the relationships between your client and community systems?
- What community systems could potentially improve your client's life?

CONCLUSION

According to Epstein and Borrell-Carrio (2005), "the clinician must adopt two types of vision—first, a direct vision of the problem unencumbered by categories, and second, a peripheral vision that can fix on relevant data at the edges of the principal focus" (p. 429). The information in this chapter is intended to strengthen your peripheral vision so you can become attuned to the critical contexts of your clients' lives, including the multigenerational family, the family's development over time, and the family's interaction with the community. This peripheral vision will be helpful with individuals, families, and, as you will see next, couples.

CHAPTER 11

Assessing Couples

Brad and Angela are both 42 and have been married 6 years. They have two children, Jackson, 4, and Samantha, 2. Angela is in tears as she relates the problems that the couple has had in recent years. She complains that they seem to be arguing over everything and are unable to communicate effectively. Both deny any domestic violence. Angela says that things were good in their marriage the first 2 years, but they began to change after Jackson was born. She feels that Brad has become increasingly distant and spends too much time at work. Brad angrily responds that he avoids coming home because "she is always on my case and I hate the constant fights." Brad also complains that the couple is no longer intimate and that they have not had sex in over 2 months. Angela retorts that she might feel like having sex if he were around more and helped out with the housework and kids. Brad dejectedly admits that he has begun to think that divorce might be the best option for the couple, which makes Angela start to cry.

If Brad and Angela were your clients, where would you begin? What issues seem to be most salient to you? If you are like most therapists who are beginning to work with couples, you may wonder where to start with a couple like Brad and Angela. This chapter and the next will help you in working with couples like Brad and Angela. This chapter begins by describing various assessment tools that you can use when assessing couples. The remainder of the chapter outlines the key areas that you should address when assessing couple functioning, which are represented by the eight C's. The next chapter builds on general couple assessment by exploring special topics that couple therapists frequently encounter, such as infidelity, sexual issues, premarital counseling, and working with same-sex couples.

ASSESSMENT TOOLS FOR COUPLES

Assessment Instruments

Assessment instruments can provide helpful data to supplement the information you gather through clinical interviewing. Below we suggest a battery of instruments you may want couples to complete. Other instruments can be substituted or added based on your preferences.

We recommend that you include a measure of relationship quality. The Dyadic Adjustment Scale (DAS; Spanier, 1976) is a popular choice among many clinicians. Scores of 107 (Crane, Allgood, Larson, & Griffin, 1990) and 105 (Jacobson & Truax, 1991) have been suggested as cutoffs for distinguishing functional couples from distressed couples. A shorter version called the Revised Dyadic Adjustment Scale has been created (Busby, Christensen, Crane, & Larson, 1995). Other measures of marital quality also exist, such as the Marital Adjustment Test (Locke & Wallace, 1959) and the Marital Satisfaction Inventory (Snyder, 1997).

Measures of marital stability can help you assess for possible issues of commitment. The Marital Status Inventory (Weiss & Cerrato, 1980) measures what steps toward divorce the couple has taken (e.g., thoughts of divorce, consulted with a lawyer). The Marital Instability Index (Booth & Edwards, 1983) could be used as an alternative to the Marital Status Inventory.

We also suggest that you include an instrument that screens for possible psychological issues or disorders, such as the Brief Symptom Inventory (Derogatis, 1993). Given the high prevalence of depression in clinical populations, a measure of depression such as those described in Chapter 6 (e.g., Beck Depression Inventory, Hamilton Rating Scale for Depression, Zung Self-Rating Depression Scale) can also be valuable.

Finally, we recommend that you include the Conflict Tactics Scale (Straus, 1979) or the Revised Conflict Tactics Scale (CTS2) (Straus et al., 1996) to assess for possible intimate partner violence or aggression.

Communication Sample

The purpose of the communication sample is to observe the couple's communication patterns. The couple is instructed to find a topic that arouses emotions of moderate intensity, and then attempt to solve the problem on their own for 10 minutes. Couples are told to choose a problem that is around a 5 on a scale of 1 to 10, where 1 represents a trivial problem and 10 represents an extremely difficult problem. You should leave the room (assuming it is possible to observe or videotape the interaction) so as not to interfere or influence the couple's discussion.

Although communication samples are sometimes used in research, they can also provide valuable clinical information. In Gavin and Nichelle's communication sample, Nichelle did the majority of talking. She suggested several things that Gavin could do to help resolve the problem. Their dynamic in the communication sample mirrored what happened at home, where Nichelle would initiate and take charge of discussions, and Gavin would passively listen to her. After observing the communication sample, the therapist hypothesized the couple may have an overfunctioning–underfunctioning dynamic.

At the end of the communication sample, you should ask if their discussion was representative of what happens at home. Often the couple will respond in the affirmative. If the discussion went better than usual, then it may be helpful to explore what was different and use this knowledge to help the couple improve their communication.

Relationship History

A relationship history can be a powerful tool for uncovering couple dynamics (Hiebert, Gillespie, & Stahmann, 1993). A review of the courtship history, for example, can point to what drew this couple together and what sustains their bond. It can also illuminate patterns that are replicated across the couple's history.

One challenge in conducting a relationship history is deciding how much detail to collect. Conducting a thorough history may take multiple sessions, particularly for couples that have been together several years. Alternatively, you may choose to conduct a more abbreviated relationship history that focuses on the most salient events in the couple's history, such as getting married, having children, or other important transitions. For couples who have had a long and eventful history, it may be difficult to conduct even an abbreviated relationship history in a single session.

A second challenge therapists can face, especially beginning therapists, is focusing too much on events and dates, overlooking the underlying processes or dynamics. You need to be continually curious as to why the events unfolded in the way they did. Rather than simply record that the couple had an unplanned pregnancy, the curious therapist will want to know why the unplanned pregnancy occurred. Did the couple discuss ways to avoid pregnancy before becoming sexually active? If not, does it reflect a couple's conflict-avoidant style?

Table 11.1 shows important areas that can be explored during a relationship history. *Dynamic Assessment in Couple Therapy* (Hiebert et al., 1993) provides a more detailed description of how to conduct an extensive relationship history, including additional sample questions that you can ask the couple.

Individual Histories

Individual histories can be an important tool in a couple's assessment, revealing historical factors that may influence their relationship. These experiences may be from one's family of origin or previous relationships. Helen recognized that neglect from her parents left her vulnerable to feeling abandoned if her husband became distant. Assessing an individual's history in a number of different areas (e.g., school, work, previous relationships) can also uncover psychopathology that may have gone unrecognized. For example, one therapist discovered that the husband had undiagnosed ADHD, which had seriously impacted his marriage.

An individual history for the purposes of couple therapy can include a number of elements. You should explore each person's family of origin, since it can influence current relationship functioning. A previous history of child sexual abuse, for example, may impact an individual's ability to be sexually intimate with his or her partner. Important beliefs about relationships or marriage can be learned from parental modeling. One man who was cohabitating with his partner stated he did not believe that marriage was either desirable or viable after watching his mother marry six different men. Another man observed how his father was "whipped" in his marriage and vowed not to let something similar happen to him. Not surprisingly, this husband was resistant to any

TABLE 11.1. Conducting a Relationship History

Relationship area	Sample questions
Attraction and mate selection	"What was your first impression of your partner?" "What did you like about your partner after the first date? Second date?" "How did your impressions change over time?"
Bonding and sex	"Who initiated the first date?" "Who took primary responsibility for initiating or planning dates?" "What types of activities did you do when dating?" "What types of activities did you do after marriage? After children arrived?" "How was physical affection displayed?" "When did you become sexually active as a couple?" "Who typically initiates sexual activity?" "How frequently did you have sex at this point in the relationship?" "Did you ever argue over sex in your relationship?" "Did sexual frequency change after any important events (e.g., getting married, pregnancy, affair)?"
Triangulation	"What role do the parents or in-laws have in your relationship?" "How does work outside the home impact the relationship?" "Do you feel your partner has ever been overinvolved with work, hobbies, family, or friends?" "Have there been any affairs? If so, how was it resolved?"
Power and autonomy	"How did you decide to set up your finances (e.g., separate or joint accounts)?" "How were major financial decisions made (e.g., buying a house)?" "How were decisions made to relocate or move?"
Conflict	"When did you have your first fight, and what was it over?" "How did you make up after the first fight?" "Did the fight change how you looked at your partner or the relationship?" "Did you have much conflict during your courtship? Early marriage?" "What issues do you generally have conflict over?" "At its worst, how bad has the conflict gotten?"
Commitment	"When did you decide to date each other exclusively?" "At what point did you begin to think of marrying your partner?" "Who first suggested or mentioned the possibility of getting married? How did the other respond?" "Were there any unplanned pregnancies prior to marriage? How did it influence your plans to get married?" "Have there been any separations? How did you get back together?"
Character features	"What did you find different or strange about your partner when you first met him (or her)?" "What did you later find different or strange about your partner as you got to know him or her better?" "What did your family and friends think of your partner?" "Have you ever worried about your partner's use of alcohol or drugs?"

(continued)

TABLE 11.1. *(continued)*

Relationship area	Sample questions
Life cycle	"How did your relationship change after you moved in together?" "How did your relationship change after you got married?" "How did things change in your relationship once children arrived?" "How were decisions about child care made?" "Were there any disagreements over parenting?" "How did things change in your relationship after children left home?" "How did things change when your partner retired?" "Have either of you experienced the death or serious illness of a parent? If so, how has it impacted the relationship?"

attempts by his wife to influence him. Self-esteem issues or difficulties with separation or individuation can also be uncovered through exploring an individual's family of origin experiences.

A brief academic and occupational history for each person can help you evaluate an individual's overall level of functioning. When doing the history, listen for possible strengths and resources that can be tapped into for couple work. Also pay attention to individuals who have struggled academically or occupationally since it may be a clue to some type of disability (e.g., learning disability), substance abuse, or psychopathology (see Chapter 6). Has the client been diagnosed with a mental illness? If so, is it being properly treated or managed? Has the individual ever attempted suicide (which may indicate a higher risk for suicide in the future)? You also need to explore the client's history of using substances (e.g., alcohol, drugs), and be alert to any possible clues that the individual is currently abusing substances.

Finally, you will want to explore each individual's previous relationship history. Do you see any relationship patterns that are being replicated in the current relationship? Have critical events from previous relationships shaped how a partner behaves in the current relationship? Individuals who have had one or more partners commit infidelity, for example, may be mistrustful of their current partner. It is also helpful to note the length and number of intimate relationships or marriages that the client has had. Has the individual, for example, ever been in a committed relationship of any substantial length prior to this relationship? How many times has the individual been married previously?

Since individual histories are typically done without the other partner present, therapists must carefully think through how they will handle confidentiality before meeting with each individual alone. There is always the risk that a client will disclose a secret to you (e.g., an affair) that he or she does not want revealed to the partner. Some therapists believe that keeping secrets will undermine the therapy process, and insist on a no-secrets policy. If you adopt a no-secrets policy, you need to inform your clients before the individual sessions that you will not keep any secrets, and can, at your discretion, bring any information learned from the individual sessions into the conjoint sessions. However, others believe that a no-secrets policy may keep individuals from sharing important information that can impact therapy, such as an ongoing affair. Each therapist must decide what approach he or she believes is best.

Bograd and Mederos (1999) suggest that therapists who follow a no-secrets policy may need to modify it when it comes to domestic violence. They recommend that the victim be assured that information in the individual session will not be shared without permission (unless there is evidence that the children are being harmed by the domestic violence). Premature disclosure may put the individual's safety at risk. If the victim is reluctant to discuss the partner's violent behavior, then this may indicate that couple therapy is contraindicated.

A STRUCTURED APPROACH FOR INITIAL COUPLE ASSESSMENT

Many therapists find it helpful to follow a structured approach when conducting an initial couple assessment. The approach we describe here is compatible with many theories, and can be used with most couples. However, it may need to be modified for some couples, particularly those in crisis.

The first session is devoted to accomplishing the tasks for an initial interview (Patterson et al., 2009), which include joining with clients, handling administrative issues, setting goals, and beginning the initial assessment. The areas of assessment discussed in Chapter 3 as part of an initial interview are applicable here. At the end of the session, couples can be given a battery of instruments to complete and return at the following meeting.

The second session begins by doing a communication sample with the couple. The therapist then reviews the couple's relationship history. An abbreviated relationship history can be completed in one session, while a more thorough history may require additional sessions.

After completing the relationship history, you conduct individual histories with each partner. Sessions devoted to individual histories can also be used to assess for domestic violence. Individuals may be reluctant to disclose domestic violence in a conjoint session if they fear there will be later repercussions at home. Therefore, we recommend that you routinely screen for domestic violence during individual sessions using the guidelines discussed in Chapter 4. Some therapists prefer to do the individual histories prior to doing the communication sample and relationship history, particularly if they suspect domestic violence.

Finally, you present the results of your assessment to the couple and offer them your treatment recommendations. It is not uncommon, however, for therapists to need more time for assessment, particularly if they are unclear about the couple's dynamics or interactional cycle.

Based on the information you have collected, you need to evaluate if couple therapy would be suitable for this couple. In some cases, the clients' individual issues are so paramount they first need individual therapy before a productive course of couple therapy can begin. Conjoint therapy might also be contraindicated in some cases of domestic violence.

After you have presented your feedback and treatment recommendations to the couple, assess their reaction. Do they feel the strengths and concerns you have pointed out accurately reflect their relationship? Do they agree with the treatment recommendations? Do both partners recognize the importance of taking personal responsibility for their part in creating and solving the problems? Is the couple comfortable continuing on with treatment? Some couples reach this point in therapy and find they do not desire to work on their relationship. In some cases, a couple may agree with your conceptualization but believe they can make the necessary changes on their own.

ASSESSING COUPLE FUNCTIONING: THE EIGHT C's

To do a thorough assessment of couple functioning, you need to explore a number of different areas. Birchler and his associates (see Birchler, Doumas, & Fals-Stewart, 1999) have attempted to capture these critical areas of couple functioning through their seven C's. For the purposes of this chapter, we have added an eighth C, children. The eight C's (see Table 11.2) are a helpful mnemonic to remind therapists of the impor-

TABLE 11.2. Eight C's for Couple Functioning and Assessment

- Communication
- Conflict resolution
- Commitment
- Contract
- Caring and cohesion
- Character
- Culture
- Children

tant areas to be attentive to when evaluating couples. A nice feature of this mnemonic is that it can be used from various theoretical perspectives. It is also versatile in that it can be used with a variety of couples, including either married or cohabiting couples and same-sex couples. Furthermore, we have found that the eight C's provide a nice framework for presenting feedback to couples on areas of growth and strengths.

Communication

Good communication skills are necessary for a couple to handle the inevitable conflicts that arise in all intimate relationships. Nearly all couples report communication difficulties when presenting for couple therapy. How does one evaluate a couple's ability to effectively communicate?

A simple but powerful model for understanding communication is illustrated in Figure 11.1. In this model, the speaker decides what the intended message is, and then sends or articulates that message using words and/or nonverbal communication. The listener must first attend to and receive the message, and then effectively decode or translate its meaning. Understanding these four steps can be the basis for evaluating a couple's communication skills.

In the first step of the speaker role, individuals vary on how clearly thought out the message must be before it is articulated. Individuals who are external processors will begin to articulate their message before it is completely formulated. Talking helps them further process their thoughts and feelings. As they continue to talk, they are constructing new drafts. In contrast, internal processors will generally not articulate what they are thinking or feeling until they have arrived at the final

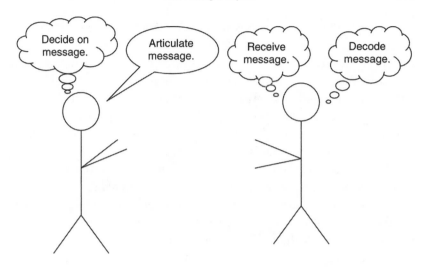

FIGURE 11.1. Basic model of communication.

draft. These individuals are often reticent to talk until they have figured out exactly what they want to say.

Couples with these two different styles can experience conflict unless they know each other's style. An internal processor may perceive that what the external processor just said contradicts something he or she said earlier. The internal processor does not recognize that the external processor is still processing things and has not arrived at the final draft. The internal processor can also be frustrated by the external processor's need to talk things out before the internal processor has had time to think through things. Conversely, the external processor may interpret the internal processor's reluctance to talk as a lack of concern for the issue or relationship. External processors can also feel out of the loop because the internal processor will not talk until he or she is able to articulate the final draft. Identifying each person's preferred style and its impact on their communication can be helpful to many couples.

A number of things can be assessed when evaluating how the speaker communicates his or her message to the partner. Gottman's research (1999) has shown that the presence of criticism, contempt, defensiveness, and stonewalling during conflict is a strong predictor of divorce. Collectively they are called the Four Horsemen. Two of these, criticism and contempt, are relevant to the speaker's role. Criticism occurs when an individual attacks a person's character or motive, such as stating, "Why don't you pick up your clothes? You are such a slob!" Contempt arises out of feelings of superiority over one's partner, and may be reflected in put-downs, sarcasm, or nonverbal behavior such as rolling one's eyes. Rather than attack the other person, the speaker will ideally state in behavioral terms what he or she is upset about and positively state what he or she needs the partner to do. This reduces the likelihood of the listener demonstrating defensiveness or stonewalling, Gottman's other two Horsemen (discussed below).

When partners communicate with each other, are the verbal and nonverbal messages congruent? Or, do they send mixed messages? If so, why? Does this reflect an underlying ambivalence about the issue? Or, are they reluctant to express their true thoughts or feelings to protect themselves or the feelings of someone else?

Can both partners accurately label or articulate their feelings? How does each partner handle the expression of emotions? Can they identify and express the softer or more vulnerable emotions like hurt and fear? Or, is anger the emotion that is primarily expressed?

When evaluating each partner's ability to be an effective listener, the first step is to observe if each is able to hear what the other is saying. Do both individuals show a genuine interest in what the other is saying, or do they seem preoccupied, inattentive, or disinterested? Individuals may become so focused on what they are going to say that they do not carefully attend to what their partners are saying. Some individuals shut down and cannot effectively listen to their partners when flooded, which may result in stonewalling, one of Gottman's (1999) Four Horsemen. Finally, does either partner have problems with hearing? Jean would often complain when her partner, Vance, would not wear his hearing aids, which was a source of frustration for her since he frequently did not correctly hear what she said.

You may also want to explore if individuals are giving signals that they are listening or tracking what is being said (e.g., making eye contact, asking questions, acknowledging what is being said). Gender issues can sometimes arise in this area (Tannen, 1990). Women normally make direct eye contact when listening to others, and they expect the same from others. Men, in contrast, may be engaged in a conversation yet not make eye contact.

The second part of being a good listener is accurately interpreting what the speaker is saying. Is each individual able to properly understand what the other is saying? If not, what accounts for this problem?

Do they have difficulty with comprehension in general, particularly with more abstract communication? Or, do they have "filters" that distort how messages are interpreted? Paul complained that his wife often made comments that made him question if she really loved him. Rosalie countered that Paul often misinterpreted what she said, and would have his feelings unnecessarily hurt. Paul had inherited a filter from his family of origin that made him question his lovability based on negative experiences with his mother.

In addition, are individuals able to validate what the other person is saying, even if they disagree or have a different perspective? Or, do individuals cross-blame, deny responsibility, or yes-but their partner? These are forms of defensiveness, one of the other Four Horsemen described by Gottman (1999).

Direct observation is an effective way to evaluate a couple's communication. Asking a couple to do a communication sample or observing the couple during other interactions in therapy can offer important clues regarding their communication skills.

Conflict Resolution

Couples come to therapy because their efforts to solve one or more problems have been unsuccessful. Therefore, exploring how a couple resolves conflict is an essential part of therapy.

It is important to determine which issues can trigger flooding in an individual, as well as what he or she does when flooded. Flooding occurs when individuals become physiologically aroused, showing signs such as an increased heart rate (Gottman, 1999). Flooding also leads individuals to perceive things more negatively. Couples are more likely to use the Four Horsemen of criticism, contempt, defensiveness, or stonewalling when flooded. They may even resort to using physical or verbal abuse when flooded. To prevent damage to the relationship, does the couple take a time out when one or both become flooded?

When assessing areas of conflict, it is important to distinguish which conflicts are due to resolvable problems and which ones are due to perpetual problems (Gottman, 1999). Resolvable problems, once properly addressed, are unlikely to reoccur. Perpetual problems, in contrast, continually resurface for a couple. According to Gottman (1999), 69% of all conflicts arise from perpetual problems and usually result from the partners being fundamentally different in their values or personalities. For Mike and Karen, their perpetual problem revolved

around how they responded to problems in life. Mike would often minimize or downplay problems while Karen often became anxious about
them. This created conflict for the couple. The more Mike downplayed
a problem, the more Karen argued how important the issue was. This
only led Mike to further minimize it in an effort to counteract what he
saw as Karen's overreaction. This pattern was evident in many of the
couple's conflicts, although the issue that precipitated the cycle was different each time.

Distinguishing between resolvable and perpetual problems has
implications for treatment. With resolvable problems, the focus can
be on finding a solution that fixes the problem. In contrast, perpetual
problems often require some measure of acceptance on the part of the
couple. Paradoxically, this acceptance can lead to the couple being less
distressed over the dynamic.

One of the keys to successfully treating couples is to identify and
change the problematic cycles that couples find themselves repeating
over and over again. These frequently take the form of a vicious circle
where each partner's behavior perpetuates the pattern. The distance–
pursuing cycle is a classic example. When one partner pursues the
other to obtain greater connection or closeness, the other partner withdraws because he or she feels smothered. This withdrawal, however,
only increases the first partner's efforts to seek greater closeness.

The cycle can be identified in a variety of ways. Often the couple
will reenact the dynamic in therapy, especially if one or both partners
become flooded during the session. Asking the couple to do an enactment or communication sample may also allow you to directly observe
the cycle in session.

Couples may also be able to describe the cycle through questioning. However, couples often are aware only of pieces of the pattern, and
may need help to see the whole cycle. Most individuals can comment
on what their partners do but have difficulty seeing their own role in
the process. Therefore, circular questioning may be effective in piecing
together the cycle. You might ask the husband, for example, "After you
get upset, what does your wife typically say or do?" If you have successfully identified the cycle, you will be able to connect each partner's
response into a circular pattern or vicious circle. Couples frequently
report that it is quite helpful to see the cycle laid out visually (e.g., on
paper or a whiteboard).

When mapping out the cycle, you should include the underlying thoughts or emotions that drive the couple's behaviors. Mark and Emily frequently fell into a pattern where Emily would withdraw in response to Mark's anger. Further assessment uncovered that Mark got mad when Emily withdrew because he interpreted her withdrawal as a sign that she did not care for him. It was discovered that Emily withdrew from Mark's anger because it provoked unpleasant memories of her abusive father.

Targeting the thoughts or emotions that drive the cycle is key to effectively intervening. In a distance–pursuing cycle, the cognitively oriented therapist might focus on the wife's interpretation that her husband's withdrawal means rejection rather than seeing it as his attempt to avoid conflict. An emotionally focused therapist will attend to the wife's hurt feelings in response to her partner's withdrawal. Regardless, it is important that you identify what drives each person's actions within the cycle.

It can be helpful to look for exceptions to the pattern using a solution-focused perspective. Exceptions can confirm your conceptualization of the problem cycle. In the example of Emily and Mark given above, Emily recognized that in the rare times she stood up to Mark rather than withdraw, he would calm down. This provided additional evidence that the couple's cycle had been correctly identified. Finding exceptions also gives the couple confidence that the pattern can be changed and insight on how to do it.

Also be alert to possible historical factors that may influence the couple's cycle, such as family-of-origin factors. Emily's response to Mark was heavily influenced by her previous experiences with her abusive father. Making these connections can help partners make sense of their mate's behavior, and view it with increased compassion.

Commitment

The third C in the framework is commitment. Couple therapy is more likely to be successful if both partners have a high commitment to the relationship. Unfortunately, this is often not the case. Many couples do not seek therapy until one or both partners are seriously thinking about divorce. As discussed in Chapter 3, this can present challenges in setting goals for the couple.

A variety of approaches can be used to assess commitment. One is to directly ask the client about his or her level of commitment using a scaling question, such as, "On a scale from 1 to 10, what is your level of commitment to the relationship?" If you have given your clients the Dyadic Adjustment Scale, item 32 can offer clues to a client's level of commitment. Commitment is probably sufficiently high if your client answers one of the two top choices ("I want desperately for my relationship to succeed, and would go to almost any length to see that it does" or "I want very much for my relationship to succeed, and will do all that I can to see that it does"). Other responses suggest the level of commitment may be wanting. The Marital Status Inventory (Weiss & Cerrato, 1980) is another way to evaluate commitment, which measures what steps toward divorce have been taken. Scores of 4 and above for husbands and 5 and above for wives are predictive of severe marital distress (Whiting & Crane, 2003). Clients who score at or above the cutoff should be carefully assessed for their level of commitment to the relationship.

Some individuals who come into couple therapy have passed the "point of no return" in terms of their commitment to the relationship. When Fernando and Patti came into therapy after many years of marital issues, Patti described several changes that she wanted her husband to make. As Fernando made these changes, Patti remained unchanged in her ambivalence about continuing the relationship. When this was pointed out by the therapist, Patti admitted that she did not think there were any changes that her husband could make that would convince her to stay in the marriage. It was becoming increasingly clear to her that she had already emotionally left the marriage. If therapy is persistently stuck, particularly in light of one partner's efforts to change, then this may signal that the point of no return has been crossed.

You should also assess what factors impact the level of commitment. Obviously the level of satisfaction with the relationship will be important. However, other factors such as financial considerations, religious beliefs, or concerns for the welfare of children may influence one's commitment to the relationship. The advice of family and friends as to whether to stay or leave should also be considered, as well as factors that may make leaving the relationship more attractive (e.g., having an affair). A lack of commitment may also reflect a loss of hope that the relationship can be saved. As couples develop a sense of hope, their commitment to the relationship may begin to rise.

Commitment issues can arise from events during a couple's courtship. If the decision to marry was made to legitimize an unplanned pregnancy, clients may later question if they would have married their partner without the pregnancy. Individuals who use marriage as a way of leaving their families of origin may also experience issues of commitment around marriage. One woman who admitted that she married her husband so that she could leave her abusive family later questioned whether she loved her husband and if she should stay in her marriage. In some cases, couples appear to "slide" (Stanley, Rhoades, & Markman, 2006) into marriage without making a formal decision or commitment to do so. Therefore, you should explore what factors impacted a couple's decision to live together or get married since these factors can point to possible concerns regarding commitment.

Contract

A couple's contract refers to the expectations that a couple has for one another and the relationship. Some of the expectations may be outside an individual's immediate awareness. Parts of the contract may be explicit, while others are implicit and must be inferred in order to uncover a couple's contract.

Couples can experience contract issues in a number of ways. Problems can arise for couples if the expectations have not been clearly defined. This issue is most likely to occur early in a couple's relationship as they learn more about each other.

Contract issues can also emerge if each partner has different expectations. For example, disagreement on how to balance connectedness and autonomy may create conflict for some couples. Different expectations may have been learned from their families of origin (see Chapter 9). Some couples may be in general agreement regarding their contract but have a problem in a specific area. Wayne and Iris had a conflict over whether or not to have an additional child but reported little conflict in other areas of their marriage. The consensus items on the Dyadic Adjustment Scale can help you identify possible contract issues, since it asks individuals to rate the extent to which they agree or disagree about a number of different topics (e.g., finances, housework, friends).

Couples who have worked out an acceptable contract can experience problems later on if life events or transitions require they renegotiate their contract. One wife was willing to do most of the housework while her husband was employed. However, upon his retirement, she expected he would help out more with housework, since he was no longer working. He, in contrast, argued that he did not retire so he could do housework. The birth or adoption of children is another important life transition that may require couples to renegotiate their contract. Serious physical illness or injury can also force a couple to renegotiate their contract if it prevents one individual from fulfilling the roles that he or she previously had.

Finally, couples may come to therapy if one partner has seriously breached the contract. Infidelity (see the next chapter) is a common example. Other actions, such as being emotionally unavailable during a critical event (e.g., illness, miscarriage), can also be perceived as a major breach of the contract. From an emotionally focused therapy perspective, these breaches can cause attachment injuries (Johnson, Makinen, & Millikin, 2001), which can create impasses in therapy until they are resolved. When conducting a relationship history, listen for significant events that have caused one or both partners distress and resulted in a loss of trust. If individuals repeatedly refer back to these events in therapy, then it may necessary to process them before therapy can focus on more present concerns.

Caring and Cohesion

Caring and cohesion are important elements to assess in a marriage or intimate relationship. As the name implies, caring refers to the acts that partners do to show that they care for and love one another. Cohesion reflects the sense of closeness that a couple experiences. Although they can be considered separate elements, they are also closely related and can mutually reinforce each other. Acts of caring can help build a sense of cohesion, whereas actions taken to strengthen a couple's cohesion can be seen as acts of caring. Indeed, physical and sexual affection blur the boundaries between the two.

When addressing caring, first assess if clients are making an effort to show caring behaviors toward their partner. Second, are they providing their partner the type of caring behavior that he or she expects or desires? Individuals may have different definitions of caring. Verbal and physical affection were ways in which love was shown in Evan's family growing up. As a result, Evan questioned whether Mary really loved him because she was seldom verbally or physically affectionate. Mary, in contrast, grew up in a family where individuals were not verbally or physically affectionate but did things for one another as an expression of love. Not surprisingly, Mary asked that her husband do more housework and help out more with the children as a demonstration of his love.

For Mary and Evan, differences in their families of origin contributed to their having different definitions of caring. Other factors, such as gender socialization, can also create differences. When a woman shares a problem with another female, she will typically validate the woman's feelings and may offer a similar experience of her own to demonstrate she understands. Tannen (1990) calls this type of support the "gift of understanding." In contrast, men typically offer suggestions on how to fix the problem, which Tannen refers to as the "gift of advice." These different ways of offering support can create conflict for couples. A woman may interpret her male partner's attempt to fix her problem as invalidating when all she wanted him to do was listen and acknowledge her feelings. He, in contrast, may be confused or frustrated that his attempts to help her have been rebuffed.

A couple's level of cohesion can be assessed in a number of ways. The Dyadic Adjustment Scale has a subscale that measures cohesion. Inspecting these items can help you assess where the couple is doing well or could improve. The affectional expression subscale on the Dyadic Adjustment Scale, which measures physical and sexual intimacy, can supplement one's understanding of the couple's bond. Couples can also be asked directly about their physical or sexual relationship (see the next chapter), or what types of activities they do together as a couple. These activities can take several forms, such as going on dates, doing recreational activities together, sharing hobbies, or volunteering together.

Also be alert to any change in the pattern of doing activities together. One couple reported that they enjoyed a lot of fun activities together when first dating, such as going to the beach or flying kites. After they moved in together, however, these activities stopped, to the detriment of the relationship. Resuming these "dates" was a key to improving the couple's relationship. Many couples with children also stop "dating" once children arrive due to the time and financial pressures of raising children. Over time, stopping these activities can erode a couple's closeness.

If the couple is low on cohesion, then you may need to help them identify ways to strengthen it. Activities the couple used to do (e.g., during courtship or dating) are good to consider. They could also complete the Inventory of Rewarding Activities (Birchler, 1983), which lists several pleasurable activities couples may enjoy. Items on the inventory that both individuals agree they would like to do are ideal activities with which to begin.

When evaluating cohesion, consider not only the amount of time spent together but also its quality. Indeed, some couples benefit from spending *less* time together but improving the quality of the time they do spend together. Robert and Carolyn reported conflict in their marriage increased after Robert retired. Although the couple spent a lot of time together, they seldom participated in activities outside the home that they found rewarding. The couple reported doing better after Robert became involved in some volunteer work, giving both partners more personal time to themselves. The couple also made an effort to share more "date-like" activities that were rewarding to them both.

Character

Character refers to the individual attributes that each partner brings to a relationship. These attributes can enhance or detract from the quality of the relationship. Character features that may negatively impact relationships include mental illness, physical illness, and substance abuse. Another important character feature is personality or temperament, which can be both a positive and a negative for a relationship.

Mental Illness and Substance Abuse

It is important to evaluate individuals for psychopathology or substance abuse (see Chapter 6) since this can impact the relationship. If mental illness or a substance abuse problem exists, you should assess how the couple interacts around the issue. Often you will uncover vicious circles that maintain both the problem and the relationship distress. There is evidence, for example, that depressed individuals behave and view their partner more negatively, creating relationship distress (Beach, 2003). This relationship distress, in turn, helps maintain the individual's depression.

Similar cycles can arise around substance abuse or other addictive behaviors. Peter and Amy presented in therapy because Amy gambled nearly every day, resulting in significant financial losses for the couple. Although Amy admitted the gambling was a problem, she expressed ambivalence about quitting. Peter interpreted Amy's ambivalence as a sign that she did not care about him or the marriage. Amy reported that Peter's criticism and anger toward her made her very anxious, which only heightened her desire to gamble.

If there is mental illness or substance abuse, it is important to assess each person's understanding of the disorder. Individuals may misunderstand their partner's behavior if they lack an adequate understanding of the disorder. One husband interpreted his wife's low sexual desire as a rejection of him rather than a symptom of her depression. The couple may also have different perspectives on the disorder, which can create conflict. In the earlier example, Peter felt that Amy's decision to gamble was a rationale process that one made based on the positive and negative consequences. Thus, he viewed her decision to gamble as a sign of her indifference for the relationship. Amy viewed her gambling more as a compulsion, and was frustrated that Peter did not show more compassion for her, given how difficult it was for her to stop gambling.

Chronic Illness and Pain

Chronic physical illness or pain can also affect relationships, directly or indirectly. Severe physical illness, injury, and pain can significantly impair an individual's level of functioning. As stated earlier, this may necessitate the couple renegotiating their contract. If a partner cannot work due to chronic illness, then financial struggles may create further stress for the couple. Chronic illness or pain may contribute to a mate's irritability or depressed mood, which can affect the couple's interactions. Illness or pain may also prevent the couple from sharing pleasurable activities that enhance the relationship. One couple reported they no longer had an active sex life because the woman could no longer tolerate sex due to her chronic back pain.

As with mental illness, it is important for you to assess how knowledgeable each partner is about the physical illness. Diane complained that her husband did not seem to understand how her fibromyalgia impacted her. He did not seem to appreciate how she could have good energy some days but experience fatigue on others. If she said she was not up to doing something with him, he would assume that she was using this as an excuse to avoid being with him, since she seemed to have energy for activities on other days.

Personality or Temperament

Another important area to explore within character is temperament or personality. Differences in temperament or personality can create conflict between a couple as result of their different orientations or approaches to life. These differences may be the basis for a couple's perpetual problem (Gottman, 1999) described earlier in the chapter.

A variety of approaches have been used to understand personality or temperament. In the psychology literature, five general domains of personality, labeled as the "Big Five" factors, have been identified through research (John & Srivastava, 1999). These factors are Openness, Conscientiousness, Extraversion, Agreeableness, and Neuroticism. Openness reflects an individual's openness to experiences, and can be manifested in various ways such as an appreciation for art, emotions, adventures, imagination, and ideas. Conscientiousness measures the extent to which an individual shows self-discipline, acts responsibly, is achievement oriented, and prefers planned rather than spontaneous behavior. Individuals high on Extraversion seek out stimulation through the external world, especially through interacting with people. They often have high levels of energy and positive emotions. Agreeableness describes individuals who are good-natured, compassionate, cooperative, and trustful. Finally, Neuroticism refers to an individual's tendency to experience negative emotions easily, including anger, anxiety, or depression. Various instruments exist to measure these five factors, such as the Trait Descriptive Adjectives (TDA; Goldberg, 1992), the Revised NEO Personality Inventory (NEO PI-R; Costa & McCrae, 1992), and the Big Five Inventory (BFI; John, Donahue, & Kentle, 1991).

The Taylor–Johnson Temperament Analysis (Taylor & Morrison, 2007) and the Myers–Briggs Type Indicator (Myers, McCaulley, Quenk, & Hammer, 1998) are two other instruments sometimes used by family therapists for measuring temperament. The Taylor–Johnson Temperament Analysis assesses individuals on nine different dimensions (see Table 11.3), mapping results for both partners on a graph for easy comparison.

The Myers–Briggs Type Indicator assesses individuals on four dimensions: extraversion–introversion, sensing–intuitive, thinking–feeling, and judging–perceiving. Although individuals are categorized as being one type or the other, it may be more helpful to conceptualize them on a continuum. The extraversion–introversion dimension is similar to the Extraversion factor described in the Big Five model, and the two are closely related (McCrae & Costa, 1989).

Sensors are people who focus on the here and now. They rely on facts and what can be determined from their senses. In contrast, intuitives, as the name implies, value intuition or hunches. They also relish in ideas, imagination, and future possibilities. This dimension strongly correlates with the Openness factor in the Big Five model (McCrae & Costa, 1989).

TABLE 11.3. Personality Dimensions Taylor–Johnson Temperament Analysis (T-JTA)

- Nervous versus composed
- Depressive versus lighthearted
- Active-social versus quiet
- Expressive-responsive versus inhibited
- Sympathetic versus indifferent
- Subjective versus objective
- Dominant versus submissive
- Hostile versus tolerant
- Self-disciplined versus impulsive

The thinking–feeling dimension relates to how individuals make decisions. Thinkers make decisions more objectively or analytically, basing their decisions on rules, policy, or what they see as right and wrong. In contrast, feelers tend to make decisions based on how it will affect other people's feelings, valuing interpersonal harmony in their decision making. There is a moderate correlation between the thinking–feeling dimension and the Agreeableness factor (McCrae & Costa, 1989).

Judgers like structure and organization, while perceivers like spontaneity. Judgers like to know what is going to happen in advance and thus tend to create and follow plans. In contrast, perceivers "go with the flow" and are open to new information or changes in direction. Judgers find it difficult to play until they have their work done, while perceivers will make play a priority even if the consequence is being pressured to meet a deadline. This dimension is moderately correlated with the Conscientiousness factor (McCrae & Costa, 1989).

These four dimensions have been used to help explain patterns in mating, parenting, and other areas (Keirsey, 1998; Kroeger & Thuesen, 1988). As the following case illustrates, identifying personality differences can further a couple's understanding of one another.

Thomas and Erin came into therapy because Thomas said he was fantasizing about having an affair. He was worried whether his wife really cared about him because she was often doing chores rather than spending time with him. When she was not doing chores or errands, she would read a book or spend time in the garden. Erin complained she had too much work to do, and when she had the rare occasion to relax, she enjoyed doing quiet activities. Thomas also wanted his wife to take more initiative in setting up social events with other couples.

Erin offered that Thomas seemed to enjoy spending time with other couples more than she did.

An assessment of each individual's personality profile using the Myers–Briggs revealed Thomas was a strong extravert and perceiver, while Erin was a strong introvert and judger. These differences in temperament were contributing to the couple's problems. As a judger, Erin had a difficult time playing or relaxing with Thomas until she felt all of her tasks were done. Due to her long list of responsibilities, Erin often felt drained by all the day's activities and chores. Like other introverts, she required solitary activities to get her batteries charged. Thus, Erin's behavior reflected her temperament rather than a lack of caring for Thomas. Thomas was told if he wanted more play time with Erin, then he would need to help more with household tasks so she did not feel as pressured or drained. Thomas agreed to do this. Erin was instructed to let go of some of her responsibilities and make time for playing with Thomas more of a priority for both her and Thomas's enjoyment. Since Thomas was the extravert, he was encouraged to take more responsibility for setting up social events for the couple.

Many of the instruments for measuring temperament are long, which may discourage routine use of them. However, if you are familiar with various dimensions of temperament, then you may be able to identify areas where the couple's personalities are significantly different even without administering an instrument. In addition, if you describe both ends of the continuum, couples may also be able to self-identify their personality type.

Values and Beliefs

Differences in values or beliefs can create conflict for couples. Couples may have different values, beliefs, or attitudes about a number of different topics, including religion, money, parenting, and politics. Arguments over finances, for example, may arise when one partner frugally saves money to ensure future security while the other spends money more liberally to enjoy life in the present. When a couple is struggling with different values or beliefs, it is sometimes helpful to identify from where those values or beliefs came. Ryan became more accepting of Monica's "excessive" concerns over how money was spent when he learned her father had gambled, often resulting in the family having to live without basic necessities.

Strengths

Although character features can present challenges for couples, it is equally important to look for strengths within this domain. For example, sharing a common set of spiritual beliefs can be a resource for a couple struggling with a crisis. Ironically, the character features that couples present as problems in therapy may have initially attracted them to one another. The judger who now sees the perceiver as irresponsible may have been initially drawn to the perceiver's fun-loving and spontaneous spirit, something that the judger wishes he or she had more of. Thus, differences in temperament or personality offer the potential for partners to complement each other. Strengths can also be found under challenging conditions. Sometimes when both partners have a mental illness, each has compassion for the other because they both know firsthand what it is like to struggle with these conditions.

Culture

Differences in cultural background are another powerful factor that can influence couples. Although differences in race or ethnicity are obvious examples, cultural differences can be more broadly defined to include other aspects, such as religious background or socioeconomic status. Some have even argued that men and women are "cultural strangers" due to the different ways they are socialized to see and act in the world (Tannen, 1990).

Several aspects should be explored when examining cultural differences. First, to what extent does the couple see their different cultural backgrounds as problematic or as a strength? Couples who have difficulty identifying strengths may need help in seeing how their cultural differences can enrich the relationship.

Second, you should determine how knowledgeable they are about each other's cultural background. Have they taken the time to learn about each other's cultures? What prior exposure, if any, have they had to the other's culture? Do they have a good understanding as to what they share in common, in addition to the differences? If they speak different languages, has each attempted to learn the other's language?

Third, does the couple perceive that cultural differences are contributing to the presenting issues? Some couples know that cultural issues play a role in their problems and may even come into therapy with this being the presenting issue. John and Paloma sought out help because of difficulties in their communication. The couple had met in Peru when John, an American, visited the country. John spoke very little Spanish and Paloma spoke very little English. When they met, her sister, Carla, who spoke English, helped to translate and bridge the gap between them. The couple came to the United States with Paloma on a student visa. Her sister remained in Peru. In addition to their language differences, John and Paloma found they had "misunderstandings" in regard to money, intimacy, and how they spent their time with friends. Their frustration mounted over their inability to solve the problems and their difficulty talking about them.

Other couples may overlook how cultural issues are impacting their relationship. This may be especially true when clients are not very knowledgeable about their partners' cultural background. You may need to help couples see how the larger cultural context shapes each person's behavior. This, in turn, may help depersonalize some of the conflict between the couple. Jacqueline, an American woman, married Juan, who was originally raised in Mexico. At the birth of their first child, Juan and his mother both assumed that Juan's mother should come from Mexico and stay with the couple for 2 months. Both believed that this was supportive and would be welcomed by Jacqueline. However, this was a source of conflict for the couple, since Jacqueline felt that her competence as a new mother was being questioned. She also felt that the privacy of their new family was being violated, and she feared that the presence of her mother-in-law in the home would interfere with Juan's ability to bond with the baby.

Gender socialization is often overlooked in couples as an important context for understanding a partner's behavior. Men and women have important differences in communication styles (Tannen, 1990), which can lead to misunderstanding between the two sexes. As stated earlier, men and women have different ways of offering support. Men and women may also look at the same set of events from different perspectives because of gender socialization. Women are primarily oriented toward interpreting relationships in terms of closeness or distance. In contrast, men are primarily oriented towards viewing relationships in terms of hierarchy and want to avoid being in a one-down position relative to others. These different perspectives can lead to conflict in heterosexual couples. Elaine, 63, would wait with anticipation for her husband, Edward, to come home from work. Upon his arrival, she would ask him questions about his day. Elaine's questions were a bid for closeness, an attempt to start a conversation with her husband. Edward, however, resented the questions because they made him feel like his wife was checking up on him, much like his mother had when he was a child. This led him to withdraw rather than respond positively to her bid for connection.

You also need to assess how cultural factors might impact the couple's interaction with their environment (Birchler et al., 1999). For some individuals, marrying someone from a different culture can create strain or a lack of acceptance from their family of origin. Thus, it can be helpful to ask how family members view the couple, and what concerns they may have expressed about the couple. Parents, for example, may fear that their adult child will change religious affiliation or drift away from religious practice if he or she marries someone outside their faith (Williams & Lawler, 1998).

Children

The eighth C in the framework is children. Children can impact marriages in a number of ways, some positive and some potentially negative. You should first inquire if the couple has children. If they do not, is that by choice, or has infertility been an issue? Infertility can place a significant stress on couples and may even precipitate the couple seeking out help. Couples can also experience secondary infertility, the inability to have a desired child after having one or more children.

If the couple has children, then it is appropriate to explore whether they are experiencing any conflict over parenting. Gerta and Jerrod described a recent conflict that had occurred with one of their children. Jerrod asked their 10-year-old son, Sean, to take out the trash. Sean complained that it was normally his brother's job and it wasn't fair for him to have to do it. Jerrod got angry with Sean, raised his voice, and threatened to take his cell phone away if he didn't take out the trash immediately. Gerta overheard the yelling and told Jerrod that he should leave Sean alone and that she would take out the trash. Jerrod stormed out of the room. In discussing this incident, the couple identified this as a common pattern they get stuck in. Jerrod wants to solve the problem quickly and easily becomes impatient. This results in him becoming harsh with the children. When Gerta perceives Jerrod as attacking the children, she becomes protective and comes to their rescue.

Conflict over parenting can arise in different ways. As illustrated above, couples may argue over one parent being too lenient or too harsh. Parents can also be criticized for not investing enough time and energy in parenting, or for being too involved in the child's life. Couples in remarried or blended families commonly struggle with defining parenting expectations, particularly around the stepparent's role (Bray, 2008).

The emotional and time demands of raising children can also affect a couple's relationship. Raising children can divert time and energy away from the marriage or relationship, reducing the couple's closeness or cohesion. This can be especially true if any of the children have special needs. Other stressors associated with parenting can also affect a couple's relationship. Terry and Brenda faced a number of stressors in their life, including a son who required a potentially life-threatening surgery to address a medical issue. The anxiety the couple faced with their son's health issues and upcoming surgery placed an additional stress on an already fragile relationship.

Children can also be triangulated into the couple's dynamics. Couples may focus on a child's problem as a way of avoiding conflict in their own relationship. Or, a parent may develop a coalition with the children against the other partner. A child may act out as a consequence of being triangulated into the marital conflict. Therefore, consider not only how children impact the marriage or couple relationship, but also how children are affected by what is going on in the couple's relationship.

CONCLUSION

In this chapter we have discussed various assessment tools that are helpful in evaluating couples, including how they can be integrated into a structured approach to couple assessment. Since couples can present many types of issues, therapists learning to work with couples can easily get lost. The eight C's, presented in this chapter, offer a useful mnemonic to guide you in your assessment of couples. Clinicians working from a variety of perspectives can use this framework to systematically assess important aspects of couple functioning. The simple and intuitive nature of the eight C's also makes them a good framework for presenting feedback to couples.

CHAPTER 12

Special Topics
in Couple Assessment

Dave nervously approaches the waiting room to meet Mark and Diane for the first session. The intake form states that they have been married 10 years and are seeking couple therapy to address an affair Mark had 6 months ago. The intake form also indicates the couple has had ongoing struggles with their sexual relationship, which deteriorated even further after the disclosure of the affair. Since this is Dave's first case with an affair, he is unsure as to what key issues he needs to address. He has little experience dealing with sexual issues, and anxiously wonders how to do a proper assessment in this area. These and other questions begin to swirl in his mind as he steps into the waiting room.

Perhaps you are like Dave, wondering how to deal with issues like affairs or sexual problems. This chapter explores assessment around infidelity and sex, two challenges therapists commonly face when working with couples. In addition, we examine assessment with two special populations, premarital couples and same-sex couples.

SEXUAL ISSUES IN COUPLE THERAPY

Sexual problems are an issue that couples encounter all too often. Therefore, you need to explore the couple's sexual relationship. For some couples, sexual problems will be the presenting complaint, while it may be part of a larger constellation of problems for others. Table 12.1 lists the sexual disorders that you as a therapist should have some knowledge of when working with couples. Following the guidelines below can guide you in your assessment of sexual issues.

Avoid the "Don't Ask, Don't Tell" Mentality

You need to recognize that many clients will be reluctant to bring up sexual issues even if they are a significant concern. Often an important clue that sexual problems exist can be found on inventories that clients fill out. For example, the Dyadic Adjustment Scale asks the extent to which the couple has disagreements over their sexual relationship, or if they have had a disagreement in recent weeks regarding being too tired for sex. It is also helpful to ask the couple directly if they experience any problems with their sexual intimacy. Your question may give the

---

TABLE 12.1. Sexual Disorders in the Treatment of Couples

Low sexual desire. The male or female has little or no thought of or desire for sex. In women, where sexual desire may be more responsive than innate, other motivations for sex (e.g., to achieve closeness) may also be diminished or absent (Basson, 2007).

Erectile dysfunction. Men have difficulty obtaining or sustaining an erection sufficient for sexual intercourse.

Arousal disorders in women. Women may experience either a lack of subjective arousal or physiological response (lubrication, vaginal swelling) when presented with appropriate sexual stimuli. Conversely, there are some women who experience persistent (and generally unwanted) physiological arousal without subjective feelings of arousal.

Female orgasmic disorder (anorgasmia). Anorgasmia refers to difficulty achieving orgasms. In primary anorgasmia, the woman has never had an orgasm. In secondary anorgasmia, the woman has lost the ability to achieve orgasms. Situational anorgasmia refers to the ability to have orgasms under certain conditions (e.g., masturbation) but not others (sexual intercourse).

Delayed ejaculation. The man is unable to ejaculate or has great difficulty ejaculating during sexual intercourse. In the most severe cases, the man may be unable to ejaculate even through masturbation.

Premature ejaculation. The man ejaculates prior to or shortly after beginning sexual intercourse (when he desires not to).

Dyspareunia. The woman experiences pain during sexual intercourse.

Vaginismus. The muscles in the outer third of the vagina go into an involuntary spasm that interferes with the woman being penetrated.

couple confidence that these concerns can be brought up and addressed in therapy.

It is not uncommon for beginning therapists to experience some initial discomfort asking about a couple's sexual life. Generally we are taught that sex is a private matter that one does not discuss with strangers. Yet, to effectively work with couples, you must overcome any hesitation and discomfort you have in talking about sex with clients. Confidently being able to ask about sexual concerns will help alleviate some of the hesitation clients may experience in discussing this topic themselves.

Use a Biopsychosocial-Systems Approach

Assessment from a biopsychosocial-systems perspective is necessary if you are to effectively identify underlying causes of sexual problems. In many cases, you may find that several of the factors within the biopsychosocial-systems framework are important and need to be addressed in treating the sexual disorder.

Sometimes sexual disorders have a biological basis. Therefore, a proper medical evaluation may be necessary to rule out physical problems or illness as possible causes. Diabetes can be an underlying cause of erectile difficulties or of anorgasmia in women (due to peripheral neuropathy). Cardiovascular disease can affect a man's ability to achieve erections. Nerve damage, a neurological disorder, or endocrine disorders can also cause various sexual disorders.

Many medications can also impact sexual functioning. Antidepressants, for example, can inhibit sexual desire or the ability to have an orgasm. Therefore, it is important to assess if the beginning of a sexual problem coincided with the start of any new medications. Alcohol and drug use can also cause sexual problems, such as erectile difficulties. Biological factors do not automatically exclude psychological or relational factors, which can also be contributing factors.

Psychological factors can play an important role in creating or maintaining sexual problems. Negative beliefs or cognitions regarding sex can create anxiety or inhibitions. Another common problem that clients with sexual problems can experience is performance anxiety. Preoccupation with one's performance can distract individuals from enjoying the sexual encounter, resulting in problems with arousal or having an orgasm. Depression can also impact a client's sexual functioning in ways that include reducing sexual desire.

Relational factors are important to assess for a number reasons. First, they may be the underlying cause for the sexual problem. Anger or resentment toward a partner, for example, may diminish an individual's level of sexual desire. Second, even if relational issues do not create the original problem, they may help maintain it. A woman who complains about her mate's erectile difficulties may exacerbate the problem by reinforcing his performance anxiety. Third, it is important to evaluate the impact of the sexual disorder on the couple's relationship since it may create conflict or impact a couple's sense of closeness.

Finally, religious or cultural/contextual factors can also impact sexual functioning. Religious socialization, for example, can shape an individual's view of sex, including what are considered acceptable and unacceptable forms of sexual expression. Gender socialization may play a role in a couple's sexual interactions, for example, by determining who initiates sex.

Conduct a Sexual History

A sexual history is an important tool in evaluating sexual problems. When conducting this history, you need to determine how prevalent the sexual problem has been across time and situations. Has the individual had the sexual problem throughout his or her life (lifelong, or primary), or has the problem emerged after a period of appropriate sexual functioning (acquired, or secondary)? You should also assess if the sexual problem happens across a number of different conditions (generalizable), or if it occurs only in specific situations or with specific partners (situational). Making these determinations may help you identify the underlying cause or causes. For example, physiological problems can likely be ruled out for a man who has little difficulty getting firm erections during masturbation but has erectile difficulties when engaging in intercourse with his partner.

Important beliefs about sex can also emerge during the sexual history. One man disclosed that his father beat him up when he discovered him as a young child "playing doctor" with a neighborhood girl. As a result, the man saw sex as something that was bad, which contributed to his presenting complaint of low sexual desire.

Often partners are more comfortable talking about their sexual history without the partner present. If the history is done in this manner, you need to be clear about what information will be kept private or can be disclosed in a conjoint session.

Carefully Assess Sexual Interactions

To effectively assess sexual problems, you will need to ask for specific information about the couple's sexual interactions. This will include assessing for cognitions, emotions, and behaviors during sexual interactions. For example, to properly assess premature ejaculation, you will need to ask when the man ejaculates (e.g., before or after penetration), and how long he is able to delay ejaculation after penetration. If there are erectile or orgasmic difficulties, exploring the couple's behaviors during foreplay is necessary to determine if the partners are receiving sufficient stimulation prior to intercourse. You will need to understand each person's internal experience during sex. Does either partner experience performance anxiety? What is the individual's level of arousal? Are physical signs of arousal in sync with subjective arousal? Delayed ejaculation, for example, may result from the man having a low level of subjective arousal despite having an erection (Hartmann & Waldinger, 2007). Questions of this nature may be uncomfortable for clients to answer, particularly if they have any inhibitions talking about sex. A secure therapeutic relationship, as well as asking the questions in a reassuring manner, can facilitate client disclosure of this sensitive material.

Explore Meaning

You need to assess what sex means to each person. Does it simply provide physical gratification, or is it a vehicle for emotional connection? Sex and intimacy can be easily confused. Some people desire sex in order to feel close to their partner. They see it as a confirmation of their feelings for that person. Others feel close after sex occurs. The partners may have very different experiences of what makes them feel close. When asked about how she shows her partner that she cares, one client said, "I wear really cute underwear, so he knows." Her partner did not realize this was her intention or that it had anything to do with her feelings for him. Differences in how closeness is expressed and desired may need to be explored.

You also need to assess what meaning each partner attributes to the sexual problem. Clients with sexual problems may be distressed about their sexuality. In addition, they may worry about their partner's reaction. Some individuals may fear that their partner will have an affair to compensate for the sexual difficulties in the relationship. You should also evaluate what meaning the partner attaches to the individual's sexual problem. Men may view themselves as poor lovers if their partner has low sexual desire or does not have an orgasm. In a similar manner, some women may fear they are no longer attractive to their partner if he has low sexual desire or has erectile difficulties. The meaning that each person attributes to the problem can impact how the couple relates around the sexual difficulties.

Assess If Expectations Are Realistic

You will also need to determine if your clients have realistic expectations about sex. It is not uncommon for individuals to be misinformed about sex or sexual norms. This can create anxiety about one's sexuality or competence as a lover, which may lead to performance anxiety. You may find that psychoeducation is beneficial in helping a couple to have more realistic expectations regarding sex.

Rule Out Other Disorders

Finally, you need to be aware that some sexual difficulties may mask or be caused by other sexual problems. A man who has low sexual desire may develop erectile difficulties due to his low arousal. Conversely, a man with an apparent low sex drive may be avoiding sex in order to avoid dealing with erectile difficulties. It may be difficult at times to sort through these issues. In some cases, one partner's sexual problem may be contributing to a sexual problem in the other partner. A woman may have difficulty with achieving an orgasm if her partner has problems with premature ejaculation, especially if the couple relies on intercourse as the primary means of sexual intimacy.

A detailed description of how to assess specific sexual dysfunctions is beyond the scope of this book. *Principles and Practice of Sex Therapy* (Leiblum, 2007) is an excellent resource for those interested in a more detailed discussion of assessment and treatment issues for specific sexual disorders. However, following the preceding guidelines will generally help you determine what are the most salient factors causing the sexual difficulties. This will enable you to decide if you have the necessary skills and background to treat the couple's issues, or if you should make a referral. If necessary, you can refer the couple to a therapist certified by the American Association of Sexuality Educators, Counselors and Therapists (AASECT).

INFIDELITY OR AFFAIRS

Helping couples navigate the strong emotions and issues that surround an affair can be a challenge for beginning and experienced therapists alike. A proper understanding of the affair can help couples begin the healing process. Indeed, some couples find their marriage or relationship is stronger after having successfully worked through the affair.

During assessment, you should determine the nature of the affair. Some affairs are emotional, some are sexual, and others are a combination of the two. Understanding the nature of the affair may help you discern the possible motivation behind it. An individual who feels lonely in his or her own marriage may have an emotional affair to compensate for these unmet needs. In contrast, a sexual affair (e.g., one-night stand) with no emotional involvement may reflect a different motivation. In some cases, the couple may not even agree if an infidelity has occurred. This is most likely to occur with emotional affairs, with the injured party claiming his or her partner's emotional involvement with another person constitutes an affair, while the other denies it is an affair since it did not include any sexual contact. In these cases, you may need to help the couple agree on a definition of an affair, which may or may not include sex.

It can also be helpful to get other specifics about the affair, such as how long it lasted. Was it a brief encounter, or did it last several months, or perhaps even several years? How long ago did it occur? This can help you discern where the couple is in the recovery process, or if they have become stuck in their attempts to heal. It is also important to ask how the injured partner learned of the affair. The way the affair was discovered can intensify the feelings of betrayal. It is a very different experience to have been surprised when you walked in on your partner with someone else than it is to have hired a private investigator.

It may be helpful at times to learn something about the person with whom the individual had an affair. This may give you clues as to why the affair happened. In fact, injured partners will often compare themselves to the "other woman" or the "other man" in an attempt to discern why the affair occurred. Often they will ask themselves, "What does he (or she) have that my partner found desirable that I do not offer?" Some individuals make comparisons based on physical attractiveness. One woman, for example, suspected that her husband was drawn to a particular woman because she had large breasts. In reality, the primary factor that contributed to his having the affair was the boost to his ego from being able to attract a younger woman.

You should also note the importance that each attaches to the affair, which is sometimes dependent on its nature. Some injured partners will be more distressed by an emotional affair (or the emotional component of a sexual affair), whereas others will be more distressed by their partner having sex with someone else. In some cases, the individual having the affair will attempt to minimize the importance of the affair based on its nature. An individual may claim that it was a one-time mistake (e.g., one-night stand), or state it was simply about sex and did not reflect love or an emotional attachment to the other person.

Also explore if there is a previous history of affairs, or if it is an isolated incident. If the couple has a chronic history of affairs, then inquire if there is something unique about this affair that prompted them to seek therapy. A chronic history of affairs may reflect a number of possible factors, including feeling entitled or justified in having an affair, a sexual addiction, or a personality disorder (e.g., antisocial). It may also be a clue to bipolar disorder, with sexual indiscretion shown during manic episodes.

With couples who have experienced infidelity, you need to assess for possible issues of harm, particularly the risk of suicide. Injured parties can experience intense feelings of distress from the betrayal, which can result in depression and suicidal ideation. The individual who committed the infidelity may also be suicidal or depressed. Often these individuals feel intense guilt, particularly after witnessing the distress their partner feels. They may also feel sadness over the affair ending, especially if they had a strong emotional connection with this person. Or, they may worry their mate will leave or end the relationship, which is a realistic concern. You also need to assess for possible physical violence, since arguments around affairs can escalate. In addition, be alert to possible threats of serious harm (e.g., against the lover).

Your assessment should include what steps the couple has taken to heal or recover from the affair. The key tasks that couples must complete can be summarized by the six A's listed in Table 12.2, which provides a nice framework for both assessment and intervention. First, assess if an apology has been made. During one therapy session, the husband said to his wife he was sorry he had been unfaithful. She turned to the cotherapists and stated that this was the first time he had put into words

TABLE 12.2. Six A's for Addressing Affairs

- Apology[a]
- Accept responsibility
- Acknowledge how the person was hurt[a]
- Atonement[a]
- Answer why the affair happened
- Accumulate trust

[a] Proposed by D. Ball (personal communication, June 17, 2009).

that he was sorry. If an apology has been made, how did the individual do it? Did his or her partner believe it was genuine? If not, why?

For the apology to be effective, it must include the next three elements on the list. The person who committed the infidelity must be able to *accept responsibility* for the affair instead of minimizing or disowning responsibility for the affair or even blaming their partner ("If you had sex with me, I wouldn't need to find it somewhere else!"). The individual must also be able to *acknowledge how the partner has been hurt.* This step must go beyond simply stating they know their partner is hurt, and requires that they articulate the various ways in which they have hurt their partner. One woman felt her husband showed a lack of respect for her by having an affair. She could not forgive him until he could see and acknowledge this. It may take time to fully uncover all the ways in which a partner has been hurt by an affair.

Atonement is the third ingredient to an effective apology. Atonement refers to the actions individuals will take to live out their apology. What steps or changes have they made, for example, to make sure they will never have another affair?

Rebuilding a relationship after an affair requires the couple to *answer why the affair happened.* Many couples cannot fully heal until they answer this question. The search for answers can sometimes create a vicious circle that can exacerbate the distress around the affair. The injured party may continually ask his or her partner questions with the goal of trying to understand why the affair happened. The person who had the affair may be reluctant to answer the questions for a variety of reasons, including wanting to avoid the partner's wrath, to protect the partner from hurt feelings, or to avoid his or her own guilty feelings. This avoidance, however, makes the injured partner even more distressed and adamant that the other disclose details surrounding the affair. Thus, a pursuer–distancer pattern can arise and complicate the healing process.

Often the explanation of why an affair happened defies a simple answer, and involves several factors. Many times, a combination of individual and relational factors have made the relationship vulnerable to an affair, as evident in the case below. Nevertheless, it is important that the clinician (and couple) be clear that responsibility ultimately rests with the person who had the affair, even if the relationship is a contributing factor. An individual has other options besides having an affair to address dissatisfaction in a relationship.

Rosauro and Elizabeth, a Filipino couple who had been married for 21 years, came in to therapy because of an affair Rosauro had recently had with another woman. Rosauro had returned to the Philippines for an extended visit with his relatives while Elizabeth and their children remained behind. During his visit, he met a young woman and began to socialize with her. He quickly became romantically involved with her, and even helped her set up an apartment where they could live. Elizabeth discovered the affair after 2 months and gave him an ultimatum to end the affair and return home, or she would divorce him. Rosauro, faced with the threat of his marriage ending, stopped the affair and returned home. In therapy, Rosauro reports he loves his wife, but has a difficult time stating why he got involved in the affair.

A number of factors seemed to contribute to Rosauro's affair. His initial involvement with the young woman was motivated out of loneliness for social interaction. He became flattered by this younger woman's attention, which made him feel good about himself. Due to self-esteem issues, Rosauro was particularly vulnerable to needing and desiring attention from this woman. Cultural factors also appeared to play a role. The couple described how it was not uncommon for affluent men in the Philippines to have mistresses. They explained that young women from impoverished backgrounds might seek out such men as a means of improving their lives. Rosauro admitted this was likely the woman's motive for the relationship, yet he had a difficult time saying no to her requests. In addition, he felt powerless to end the relationship even though his feelings of guilt began to grow. It was only the threat of divorce that finally compelled Rosauro to end the affair. Elizabeth acknowledged Rosauro had great difficulty setting limits and saying no to others. She often felt he would help others yet was unwilling to stand up for her needs, particularly if they conflicted with the needs of his family. This had been a source of chronic conflict in their marriage. Through therapy, he began to recognize he had a difficult time saying no to others because of a fear of rejection. However, he always believed Elizabeth would love him no matter what, leading him to ignore her needs and take her for granted. It was only after her threats to divorce him that he realized he could lose her.

Answering why the affair happened can further a client's progress in addressing the other A's. Rosauro started becoming more assertive in setting limits with his family of origin and standing up for Elizabeth's needs. Being more assertive in this manner was part of his atonement, the process of living out his apology. Elizabeth, recognizing how difficult this was for Rosauro, began to trust his commitment to the marriage.

Another challenge couples face is to reestablish or *accumulate trust*. Establishing trust can be conceptualized in two parts. First, the injured partner needs to feel confident the affair has ended. It is not uncommon for the injured party to doubt the affair is completely over. In some instances, this fear is justified because the affair is continuing. Therefore, assess the extent to which the injured partner's fears seem legitimate. Second, the injured partner needs to feel confident an affair will not happen again. Couples who have been able to successfully uncover why the affair happened generally feel more confident in their ability to prevent future affairs.

Accumulating trust is a process that takes time. You should explore with your couple what efforts are being taken to build trust. Is the person who committed the affair sensitive to the partner's fears? Is the individual being transparent regarding his or her whereabouts and actions, or is he or she being secretive? Is the injured party checking up on the partner (e.g., reading e-mails)? How does the partner respond to this? Is this seen as a violation of privacy, or a necessary part of building trust? It may also be important to explore what happened around the disclosure of the affair. If the individual denied the affair when initially confronted, that may make it more difficult for the injured partner to believe in his or her honesty.

PREMARITAL COUNSELING

A special population that you may encounter is the engaged couple preparing for marriage. It is important to consider how a premarital couple presents in therapy. Some couples come to therapy because they are already in distress. In these circumstances, work will proceed in a similar manner to work with other couples where the goal is to alleviate distress. Some couples, however, come to make sure they are adequately prepared for their forthcoming marriage. In these cases, the focus is more on prevention than intervention, although some couples require elements of both.

The eight C's described in the previous chapter can provide an effective assessment framework for engaged couples. The importance of *communication* and *conflict resolution* skills is evident from the fact that many premarital programs such as PREP, Couple-Communication, and Relationship Enhancement (Williams, 2007) focus on teaching couples these skills.

Although engaged couples typically have a high *commitment* to the relationship, one should assess if there are any issues that might undermine their future commitment. For example, did the couple feel pressure to get married due to an unplanned pregnancy? Does the couple have realistic expectations about married life? Couples with an overly idealistic view of marriage may become disillusioned when some of the excitement inevitably fades, and may question whether they should have married.

In terms of *contract*, engaged couples may still be discovering what each other's expectations are. Premarital inventories (discussed below) can help couples uncover their expectations. Couples can also experience problems negotiating what the marriage will be like. Each person has a blueprint for how it should be built, and if the couple is not careful, they can develop a power struggle over its design.

The remaining C's—*caring, character, culture,* and *children*—are also worth exploring with engaged couples. Does each partner, for example, understand the other's preferred style of caring? Do they recognize how differences in personality or values may be impacting the relationship, creating the potential for conflict? You should also screen couples for substance abuse and physical aggression. Is the couple effectively managing cultural differences? If they are bringing children into the marriage from previous relationships, carefully explore if they have realistic expectations about blended families and have worked out a reasonable plan for dealing with parenting issues that can arise (Bray, 2008).

Since the majority of premarital counseling is done in a church context (Stahmann & Hiebert, 1997), you will need to be comfortable assessing and discussing spiritual issues. In fact, *church* could be added as a ninth C to the framework to represent the need to examine religious or spiritual issues. You will want to examine how the couple's spiritual beliefs and practices will shape the marriage in regard to issues such as gender roles or family planning. Religious differences may be another important consideration, since they can create the potential for conflict (e.g., disagreement over the religious upbringing of children) or make it more difficult for a couple to form a religious or spiritual bond. Problems can also exist between partners who belong to the same denomination or religion, particularly if there are significant differences in religiosity. Finally, you may want to explore if the couple participates in a religious community, since this may be an important part of their social support network.

Many of the assessment tools discussed in the preceding chapter can be applied to premarital couples. Doing a relationship history with premarital couples can be an effective way to uncover couple dynamics. Many couples find this an enjoyable and nonthreatening way to explore their relationship (although some may present with a conflictual history).

Experiences from one's family of origin can strongly shape one's expectations and behaviors within marriage. Thus, many premarital counselors like to explore each partner's family of origin (e.g., Stahmann & Hiebert, 1997). Constructing a genogram (see Chapter 10) is often an effective means of uncovering and beginning a discussion of these influences.

Premarital inventories are an important and widely used assessment tool in premarital counseling. The three most widely available and empirically tested instruments are PREPARE, FOCCUS, and RELATE (Larson, Newell, Topham, & Nichols, 2002). Individuals who do premarital counseling should become familiar with one or more of these inventories. PREPARE (*www.prepare-enrich.com*), FOCCUS (*www.foccusinc.com*), and RELATE (*www.relate-institute.org*) all have websites for learning more about these instruments.

These inventories are intended to help the couple explore the strengths and possible areas of growth in their relationship. Communication, conflict resolution, personality, finances, sex, leisure, religion and values, and family and friends are examples of topics addressed by the inventories. There are also questions that flag potentially serious concerns such as physical aggression or substance abuse.

Premarital inventories are not intended as tests used to evaluate whether a couple should get married, although some couples decide not to marry after reviewing the results. Rather, the instruments are supposed to facilitate a process of dialogue and discovery about the relationship. Two of the inventories, PREPARE and FOCCUS, require facilitators to administer the instrument and to provide the couple feedback based on the results. RELATE, however, can be taken independently by a couple, although they may still benefit from someone going over the results with them.

One challenge you may face when doing premarital counseling is the couple's reluctance to admit problems exist. This can be due, in part, to an idealistic view of the relationship. Some couples may be nervous about admitting they have problems. Identifying and acknowledging the couple's strengths, in addition to possible growth areas, can reassure them. Normalizing the fact that all couples have areas for growth can also help alleviate their fears. Finally, couples may need reassurance that your job is not to tell them whether or not they should marry, but simply to give them insight and tools for making their relationship successful.

SAME-SEX COUPLES

The eight C's for couples presented in the previous chapter are good areas to address for both heterosexual and same-sex couples. However, Green and Mitchell (2008) note that there are three special challenges that same-sex couples may face: coping with minority stress, resolving relational ambiguity, and building a cohesive social support network.

Unlike heterosexual couples, same-sex couples can face prejudice, discrimination, and marginalization due to their sexual orientation. Gay or lesbian individuals can internalize these negative or anti-gay attitudes. The combination of external and internalized sources of prejudice ("minority stress") can manifest itself in the couple's relationship in a number of different ways (Alonzo, 2005; Green & Mitchell, 2008). The partners may find themselves in arguments as a result of frustration displaced upon the partner. Sexual problems (e.g., low sexual desire) can also arise due to guilt or inhibitions. Or, depression or withdrawal from a partner may result from feeling unworthy or ambivalent about committing to a same-sex relationship. Therefore, you should assess the degree to which the couple struggles with minority stress. Where do individuals experience discrimination or prejudice due to their sexual orientation? To what extent do they struggle with self-esteem as a result of internalized negative attitudes about being gay or lesbian? Is there any evidence minority stress is contributing to relationship difficulties?

Relational ambiguity is another potential challenge facing same-sex couples since they do not have a legally and socially endorsed framework for being a couple (Green & Mitchell, 2008). Relational ambiguity may manifest itself in a number of different ways, including a struggle with "ambiguous commitment." As a result, it may be important to explore with the couple their perceptions of their commitment. Do they see their relationship as a lifelong commitment? Have they had some form of a ceremony to express this commitment? To what extent do they see themselves as responsible for the other's care in the event of illness, injury, or disability? If they view themselves as being in a lifelong committed relationship, have they taken appropriate legal steps, such as writing a will or obtaining a health care power of attorney? Some same-sex couples need to negotiate whether the relationship will be sexually exclusive or open. If the latter, has the couple agreed on the rules for having an open relationship (e.g., whom one can have sex with, what forms of sex are allowed, safe-sex practice)?

The degree to which both partners are "out" or have disclosed their sexual orientation to others can contribute to relational ambiguity. If one or both individuals have not come out, then it will be difficult for the couple to openly share with others that they are indeed a couple. The couple may be viewed as roommates or friends rather than intimate partners. Differences in being out can also create potential problems between the partners. Rita questioned Brenda's commitment to the relationship because Brenda refused to come out to her coworkers.

Gender roles can also impact same-sex couples, creating another potential source of relational ambiguity (Alonzo, 2005; Green & Mitchell, 2008). Unlike heterosexual couples, same-sex couples cannot fall back on gender-linked roles in defining the relationship. Therefore, you should examine the extent to which the couple has been able to negotiate expectations and roles within the relationship, particularly those that are traditionally gender based. For example, have they come up with a division of chores that is satisfactory to both? Are they comfortable with who initiates sex?

Assessing the same-sex couple's social support network is also important, especially since they may struggle with a lack of acceptance or marginalization due to their sexual orientation. Exploring each partner's family of origin is obviously important. Your assessment should include family members' support of the individual in general, their support of his or her sexual orientation, and their level of support for the couple's relationship (Green & Mitchell, 2008). In some cases, you may discover one or both individuals have not disclosed their sexual orientation to family members, or that they are in a same-sex relationship. Unfortunately, many gay and lesbian individuals find their families do not accept or support their sexual orientation. Even if a family does accept the individual's sexual orientation, they may not be able to fully understand (and thus support the individual).

As a result, many gays and lesbians look outside their families to find support. Sometimes individuals who provide this needed support are considered their "family of choice." Due to their importance, it is critical that you assess the couple's friendships, an area some therapists may overlook. To what extent does the couple have close friends who are accepting and supportive of their sexual orientation and relationship? This is an area that may need attention for some couples to ensure they have adequate social support.

CONCLUSION

This chapter has examined two common challenges therapists often face when working with couples: infidelity and sexual issues. The six A's can be a helpful mnemonic for evaluating a couple's progress in recovering from an affair. Using the biopsychosocial-systems model described in the first chapter is essential to identifying all the possible factors that may be causing or maintaining sexual problems. We have also offered other guidelines to help you in your assessment of sexual disorders.

In this chapter we have also looked at special considerations in working with two populations that couple therapists may treat—premarital and same-sex couples. The eight C's described in the previous chapter are useful for assessing both of these populations. However, both have unique needs or issues that need to be considered in assessment. We note, for example, that religious factors may be particularly salient in premarital counseling, suggesting the need to add a ninth C, church. For same-sex couples, we highlight the need to evaluate minority stress, relational ambiguity, and the couple's social network.

CHAPTER 13

From Assessment to Treatment (and Beyond)

I magine Tom and Maria have come to you for marital therapy. Both are in their mid-40s and have been married for 10 years. Tom is white, while Maria is Hispanic. When asked why they are coming to therapy, Maria tells you there is no passion in the relationship, which she describes as more like "brother and sister." She says there has never been much passion in the relationship, and wonders whether Tom is the right person for her. Tom tells you he has trust issues with his wife because he suspects that she has been unfaithful, although he does not know for sure. Both report stress and conflict over finances. The couple denies any physical violence. They both express doubts about remaining in the marriage.

Maria does not work outside the home, while Tom works in an administrative position that he describes as being very stressful. Maria has a number of health problems, including arthritis, fibromyalgia, migraines, and chronic foot pain. Tom complains of poor sleep. Both admit to being depressed. Tom is not currently taking any medications. Maria states she feels fine in the morning, but she then becomes depressed in the afternoon. She has been taking Wellbutrin for several months but reports no benefits from it. She also admits that she has difficulty controlling her anger. In session, she presents as energetic and has a fast-paced speech pattern. Tom, in contrast, is reserved.

When doing the relationship history, you learn that Maria had 15 months of sobriety from drugs and alcohol when the couple first met. The couple did relatively well the first few years of marriage, although they did seek out some counseling. Things changed significantly after a move to the Northeast. Tom became very involved in his career at that point and had little time for his wife. Maria compensated for this by getting involved with friends and other activities. After the couple returned to California, their problems seemed to get worse. At this point, Maria became depressed.

During her individual history, Maria reports that she was the oldest of three in her family, which resulted in her having a lot of responsibility for her younger siblings. She was molested by her father, but also has many fond memories of her family doing activities together (including with her father). Beginning in high school, Maria developed alcohol and amphetamine dependence and was sexually very active. She has been sober and clean for 13 years.

In his individual history, Tom reports being raised in a very traditional home. His father worked long hours and did not have a close relationship with him. His mother did not work outside the home. He feels that his parents gave his sister more attention to support her athletics.

If you were seeing Tom and Maria, what kind of treatment plan would you follow? Most beginning therapists find developing a treatment plan a struggle. They often have difficulty taking all of their various hypotheses and shaping them into a concise and workable treatment plan. In this chapter, using Tom and Maria as an example, we describe a process to help you create a treatment focus for your cases.

Assessment, however, does not conclude once the treatment plan has been formulated. You must also assess how the client is responding to treatment. Does your treatment plan continue to make sense as you learn more about your clients? Even if you have confidence in your conceptualization of the case, you must evaluate how effective your interventions are in addressing the issues. Finally, you must be able to assess when your clients are ready for termination. These issues are also explored in this chapter.

TRANSFORMING ASSESSMENT INFORMATION INTO A TREATMENT PLAN

Developing a treatment plan requires that you take the assessment information and transform it into therapeutic goals—goals or changes you would like to see the clients work on in therapy. Therapeutic goals are different from the client goals defined in the initial interview. Client goals state what the end result should be, while therapeutic goals state what needs to change in order for the client goals to be achieved. For example, a couple's goal may be to reduce conflict and feel more connected. Therapeutic goals may include interrupting the couple's interactional cycle, reducing substance use, and increasing the number of pleasurable activities that the couple engages in together. For therapy to be successful, there must be a connection between the therapeutic goals and the client's expected outcome or goals.

Multiple factors may inform a therapist's treatment plan (see Figure 13.1). Obviously theory is an important component. Indeed, a therapist's theoretical approach both informs what questions are asked and how the information is interpreted. A transgenerational therapist, for example, will take an interest in family-of-origin influences for both Tom and Maria.

Research can be another important influence on the development of a treatment plan. Evidence-based practice encourages therapists to think about which treatments have empirical evidence supporting their effectiveness. Research can also inform our understanding of certain problems, which may shape how we conceptualize a case. When Carol began to work with Douglas, a 14-year-old boy recently diagnosed with Asperger syndrome, she surveyed the research because she lacked a strong understanding of the disorder. After reading the literature, Carol

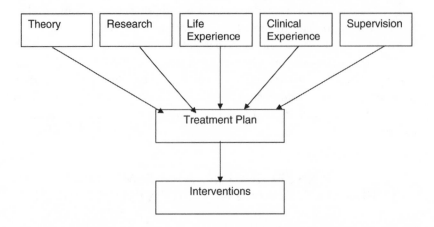

FIGURE 13.1. Factors that can influence treatment planning.

realized that she would need to help Douglas strengthen his social skills, which became a focus in therapy.

Life experience and clinical experience also inform how one conceptualizes a case. If we have had to face a challenge similar to that of our clients, we can use the knowledge we gained from our life experience to help formulate a treatment plan. Similarly, clinical experience can provide us insight into what works (or does not work) in addressing certain issues or problems. This is one reason why beginning therapists initially have such difficulty developing treatment plans. They do not have the clinical experience that more seasoned clinicians have. This is why supervision can be so important when developing a case formulation or treatment plan.

We recommend explicitly writing out each of the steps when developing a treatment plan. We have found that beginning (and experienced) therapists often benefit from this process. The steps are as follows:

- *Step 1: List problems.* In the initial step, you will list all the problems that have been identified through assessment. This will include any symptoms that have been described or observed by either the client or therapist. Listing symptoms may be important in hypothesizing about possible mental illness. Table 13.1 shows the list of problems and symptoms that could be listed for Tom and Maria, the couple presented at the beginning of the chapter.

- *Step 2: Develop and list hypotheses.* In the second step, you write down all of the most relevant and realistic hypotheses. Table 13.2 shows

---

TABLE 13.1. Step 1: Description of Problems (and Symptoms) for Tom and Maria

- Depression for Tom
- Depression for Maria (unresponsive to Wellbutrin, declining mood in the afternoon)
- Tom reports difficulty sleeping
- Health issues for Maria (arthritis, migraines, fibromyalgia, chronic foot pain)
- Financial conflict
- Maria reports marriage lacks passion
- Maria reports being bored and lonely
- Both considering divorce
- Tom reports significant job stress
- Tom suspects his wife has had an affair
- Disagreement over physical affection

TABLE 13.2. Step 2: Developing Hypotheses for Tom and Maria

- Maria has bipolar disorder (depression, cycling of moods during the day, high-energy, pressurized speech pattern, problems with anger).
- Maria's depression is due to health issues (chronic pain, fibromyalgia, etc.).
- Maria's depression is due to her marital dissatisfaction (lack of closeness in the marriage).
- Tom's complaints about sleep are due to his depression and stress.
- Tom's depression is due to work stress.
- Tom's depression is due to biological causes.
- Both partners' lack of satisfaction reflects a lack of cohesion in the marriage.
- Moving uprooted Maria from the people and activities that filled her emotional needs in the absence of her husband. Thus, her symptoms (and the marriage) worsened when the couple relocated.
- Tom is preoccupied with his job in order to gain recognition for achievement he never received in his family of origin (competition with sister for parental attention).
- Tom has allowed the couple to overextend themselves financially in order to appear successful (self-esteem issues).
- Tom has allowed the couple to overextend themselves financially in order to meet the traditional gender expectation that the husband will be a good economic provider.
- Tom's fears are legitimate because Maria did indeed have an affair, but she is afraid to admit it.
- Tom's concern that Maria has had an affair reflects his own insecurity or self-esteem issues (and not Maria having actually had an affair).
- Maria chose a nonpassionate man because she wanted someone "safe" given her history of sexual abuse. Conversely, Tom chose Maria because she was "dangerous" and would make his life more exciting.
- The couple's thoughts of divorce reflect a lack of hope, and are not an indicator that they actually want out of the relationship.

a possible list of hypotheses for Tom and Maria. At this point of the process, you may have a long list of hypotheses. This is fine, since you will be narrowing the treatment focus in the next step.

Therapists working from different theoretical perspectives may have different hypotheses, or may define the issues using different terms. When you generate a list of hypotheses, you may even find that you have included hypotheses from different theories. Since many therapists work from an integrative perspective, this does not necessarily reflect a problem.

A biopsychosocial-systems model encourages us to look at the problems from different angles. Some therapists may assume that low sexual desire is due to relational problems for the couple. Although this is a hypothesis that should definitely be considered, it is also important to be alert to the possibility that low sexual desire may be due to depression, illness (e.g., thyroid problem), or a side effect of medication (e.g., SSRI antidepressants).

When developing hypotheses, it is helpful to consider the extent to which they are descriptive or causal in nature. If you notice that a client reports irritability, difficulty sleeping, and a lack of appetite, then a legitimate hypothesis is that he or she is depressed. However, this hypothesis is at a rather descriptive level, and does not address *why* the client may be depressed. Hypotheses that are more causal in nature (e.g., the client is depressed because of low marital satisfaction) are more effective at guiding treatment.

To move from a descriptive to a more causal level, it is helpful to keep asking, "Why?" For example, start by asking, 'Why is the client depressed?" If you hypothesize that a client's depression is caused by low self-esteem, then a good question to ask is "Why does my client have low self-esteem?" You might hypothesize that your client struggles with low self-esteem due to some negative schemas internalized from his or her family of origin. Challenging these negative schemas might then be one of your therapeutic goals. Using a chain of "why" questions in this way can lead you to hypotheses that are less vague and suggest more concretely how treatment should proceed.

• *Step 3: Develop a treatment focus.* Beginning therapists are often good at generating hypotheses. Where they can get stuck is in narrowing and consolidating their hypotheses into a workable treatment plan. We strongly recommend that your treatment plan not exceed two or three therapeutic goals at any one time. Otherwise, it is too easy to lose focus and feel pulled in many directions. When it comes to maintaining a treatment focus, your mantra should be "Do more with less." Table 13.3 shows the therapeutic goals for Tom and Maria at two different stages of treatment—the preliminary and middle stages.

As Table 13.3 illustrates, the therapeutic goals will likely change as therapy evolves. As some goals are accomplished, new goals may become the focus. This may require the therapist to prioritize certain therapeutic goals over others. In the case of Tom and Maria, the therapist focused on building couple cohesion early on in treatment. The

TABLE 13.3. Step 3: Developing a Treatment Focus for Tom and Maria

Initial treatment plan	Later treatment plan
1. Build couple's cohesion.	1. Address trust cycle.
2. Rule out bipolar disorder for Maria.	2. Rebalance work/family for Tom.
	3. Improve self-care for Maria.

therapist hypothesized that this would help build a sense of hope and strengthen the couple's bond, which might make it easier for them to do the emotionally difficult work of examining trust issues. As they began to regularly go out on dates, they reported feeling better about the relationship and developed a renewed sense of hope. The therapist could now revise the therapeutic goal from building cohesion to focusing on trust issues.

The fact that therapeutic goals change over time does not mean that they keep changing from session to session. If this happens, it is usually a sign that the therapist has not developed or committed to a treatment focus. Writing down the therapeutic goals for each case and reviewing them prior to each session can help keep you on task. If you have done a good job developing therapeutic goals, you can often take the material your client brings into each session and use it to address one of your therapeutic goals.

Sometimes an initial treatment goal may reflect the need to do further work to rule out a hypothesis. In this case, the therapist suspected that Maria could be suffering from bipolar disorder based on her symptoms (e.g., cycling of mood during the day, difficulty with anger, poor response to Wellbutrin). If Maria indeed did have bipolar disorder, then she may have needed a different medication to adequately control her mood. Interventions included psychoeducation with Maria so she could assess if her experience fit with that of someone having a bipolar disorder, as well as a referral to a psychiatrist to help rule out such a disorder. It was later ruled out, which suggested that other underlying causes of depression should be targeted.

When developing a treatment focus, it is sometimes possible to combine or link multiple hypotheses into a single therapeutic goal. For example, one of the therapist's goals was to help Tom rebalance his priorities with regard to work and family. The therapist believed that in order for the marriage to improve, Tom would need to devote more time to the marriage and cut back on the time he spent at work.

Rebalancing the time he spent at work and at home would tie together several of the hypotheses that the therapist entertained. Reducing his time at work might lower Tom's stress level, perhaps alleviating his depressive symptoms. It would also likely involve looking at why Tom felt so compelled to work excessive hours, which the therapist hypothesized was due to his strong need for recognition (based on family-of-origin dynamics). Obviously, it would it also make him more available to his wife, which could reduce her sense of isolation and loneliness.

As family therapists, we attempt to understand the relational context of an individual's behavior. Thus, many of our therapeutic goals should reflect an interactional understanding as to why the problems exist. In Tom and Maria's case, the therapist eventually came to recognize how the couple's dynamics helped create and perpetuate their issues around trust. Tom's accusation that Maria had had an affair hurt her deeply, leading her to begin withdrawing from him. Her withdrawal, however, fueled Tom's insecurities about the relationship, including his suspicions that she was having an affair.

In an effective treatment plan, therapeutic goals often reinforce each other in a synergistic manner. Rebalancing Tom's work and family commitments made him more available to Maria. It also led him to become happier, not only in his marriage, but in his life in general. Furthermore, Maria found it easier to be with him since he was less depressed, which reassured him of her love. Maria learned to practice better self-care, both as a way to cope with her numerous health issues and also to make her less dependent on Tom for her emotional needs. By practicing better self-care, Maria became less reactive to Tom's moods, enabling her to stay more engaged.

ASSESSMENT DURING TREATMENT

Assessment does not end with the development of a treatment plan. As stated in the first chapter, assessment is intervention, and intervention is assessment. As you begin to intervene with clients, it is important to assess how clients respond to treatment. This, in turn, may give you a better understanding of your client and of how to intervene more effectively.

Measuring Change

As you proceed through therapy, it will be important to assess how much progress your clients are making. Measuring client progress raises the difficult question "What does change look like?" Do you need to see a change in the couple or family dynamics to consider it real change, or is elimination of the presenting problem sufficient? Is behavioral change necessary for a successful outcome? Or, can a change in perception, such as greater acceptance of the problem, also be considered a success?

Whose perception of change should take precedence? If a client believes that things are better, but the therapist has observed little change, whose perspective counts the most? Conversely, if a therapist sees changes, but the client does not recognize them, does that constitute real change? How you answer these questions will shape how you define and measure success in therapy.

We believe resolving the presenting problems and observing changes in relational dynamics are both important. Although we generally seek to change relationship dynamics, it is possible that some presenting issues can be resolved without changing couple or family dynamics. Ideally, change will be evident both behaviorally and on the perceptual (cognitive and/or emotional) level. However, we recognize how one views the problem or situation is often a powerful form of change in itself, and that behavioral change is not always present.

In general, we believe the client should be the primary authority on whether successful change has occurred. Ultimately the clients must live with whatever changes are made or not made, so we look to them to answer the question of whether their lives are better for having received our services. Still, we do not automatically discount our own perspective. We may be the first to notice the changes the client is making, and can use this to draw attention to what we want the client to continue to do. In some cases, it may be appropriate to challenge the client to make additional changes to reduce his or her vulnerability to problems reoccurring in the future.

Due to its complexity, you may want to use multiple ways of assessing change. Fortunately, you have a number of tools at your disposal. Asking clients about changes they have observed in their lives is an appropriate place to start. This can be done in a variety of ways. One might ask clients directly through open-ended questions, such as "What changes or improvements in your life/relationship have you observed?"

Clients might also be asked periodically to rate on a scale from 1 to 10 how well they are doing, and comparisons made with how they were doing before. Although clients are in the best situation to observe if changes are happening in their lives, there are potential problems of which you should be aware. Clients may be tempted to say they are doing better than they really are to look good (social desirability) or to protect the therapist's feelings (demand characteristics).

You can also use your own powers of observation to note if changes are happening. Clients who are feeling better about themselves or their relationship may have a different presence about them (e.g., lighter, less depressed affect). You may also notice that family members or partners are interacting differently within the session. These are often good indicators of change. In some cases, you may observe the changes before the client is consciously aware of them. However, it may be difficult for you to recognize change if it has occurred primarily at a perceptual rather than a behavior level.

Occasionally, clients will comment that others have pointed out changes in them. One man noted that coworkers began to ask him what was going on because they had noticed his mood was more positive. This is another powerful indicator of change. Therefore, it can be important to ask clients if others have noticed or commented on how they seem different.

Pencil-and-paper assessment instruments can also be used to measure change. If you had clients complete instruments that measure individual, couple, or family functioning as part of your initial assessment, then these instruments could be readministered later in therapy to determine if there has been change. For example, a couple who completed the Dyadic Adjustment Scale at the beginning of therapy could retake it later in the course of therapy. This could help you determine not only if the relationship has improved, but also if their scores have moved into the functional or nondistressed range.

Lambert and Hawkins (2004) recommend that clients fill out assessment instruments throughout therapy to monitor their progress rather than only at the beginning and end of treatment. If the client is not making progress early in therapy, then you can identify what factors may be barriers to change (see the following section). For brief therapy, you might consider giving the clients a weekly assessment, particularly in the beginning. For clients who remain in therapy for a longer period of time, a monthly assessment may be sufficient. Obviously, this approach is most practical if the instruments are brief and easily completed by the client. Even a brief form that asks the client if things are significantly better, somewhat better, the same, somewhat worse, or significantly worse compared to last week can help you assess if positive change is occurring.

Lambert and Hawkins (2004) recommend the BASIS-32, the Brief Symptom Inventory (BSI), and the Outcome Questionnaire (OQ-45) as outcome measures widely used in the literature and relevant to clinical use. The BASIS-32 (Eisen, Grob, & Klein, 1986) is used to assess mental health status among clients receiving psychiatric care. In addition to a total score, the BASIS-32 yields scores on five subscales—Relation to Self/Others, Depression/Anxiety, Daily Living/Role Functioning, Impulsive/Addictive Behavior, and Psychosis. The BSI (Derogatis, 1993) is a 53-item inventory that can be used to measure psychological distress. It consists of nine symptom subscales that include Somatization, Obsessive–Compulsive, Interpersonal Sensitivity, Depression, Anxiety, Hostility, Phobic Anxiety, Paranoid Ideation, and Psychoticism. It also has three global indexes, the Global Severity Index, Positive Symptom Distress Index, and Positive Symptom Total Index. Norms exist for normal, outpatient, and psychiatric populations. The OQ-45 (Lambert et al., 2004) is a 45-item scale that measures client progress in therapy, and includes three subscales that measure symptom distress, interpersonal relations, and social role functioning. The Youth Outcome Questionnaire (Y-OQ) is a version of the OQ-45 suitable for youth (Burlingame et al., 2005).

Other instruments for measuring client progress have also been developed. The Systemic Therapy Inventory of Change (STIC) can be used to track client change for adults, couples, families, or children (Pinsof & Chambers, 2009). Two forms of the STIC exist. The Initial STIC, which is administered before the initial interview, consists of six parts, which assess: (1) demographics, (2) individual functioning, (3) family-of-origin recollections, (4) couple functioning, (5) family functioning, and (6) child functioning. Clients fill out all the parts that apply to them based on their demographics. The Intersession STIC, which was developed to be administered each therapy session, typically takes clients 5 to 7 minutes to complete. The Intersession STIC includes shorter versions of the questionnaires used to measure individual, couple, family, and child functioning. It also includes brief measures that assess the therapeutic alliance between the therapist and clients in individual, couple, or family therapy.

Two other measures that are used together to measure client progress are the Outcome Rating Scale (ORS; Miller, Duncan, Brown, Sparks, & Claud, 2003) and the Session Rating Scale (SRS; Duncan et al., 2003). Both scales include only four items apiece, so they can be administered quickly. The ORS is given at the beginning of every session to measure change, while the SRS is administered at the end of each session to assess the therapeutic alliance. The Child Outcome Rating Scale (CORS; Duncan, Sparks, Miller, Bohanski, & Claud, 2006) and the Child Session Rating Scale (CSRS) are child versions of the scales, appropriate for youth ages 6–12 years. Miller, Duncan, Brown, Sorrell, & Chalk (2006) found that obtaining client feedback using these scales improved client outcomes and reduced client drop outs.

Assessing Barriers to Change

If there does not appear to be satisfactory movement in therapy, then it is important to assess what might be contributing to the lack of progress. One area to explore is the therapeutic relationship, since it is essential to the success of therapy. Have you been able to develop a strong therapeutic relationship? You should continue to monitor the relationship throughout therapy. Do you see any signs that a client feels the relationship has been damaged in some manner? Instruments such as the Intersession STIC and the SRC, described above, can help you assess the therapeutic alliance. When you are working with relational systems such as a couple or family, do all members feel that you are being balanced and/or fair when challenging or supporting individuals within the system? Or, do individuals feel that you are aligned with a particular family member? At times, individuals will state this concern directly. However, often these concerns may be addressed less directly. For example, if a parent argues that you do not see through an adolescent's manipulation, the parent may be expressing concern that you are too aligned with the adolescent.

If progress is not being made, then you may need to reevaluate whether you have a good contract for therapy. Some therapists, in their eagerness to bring about change, forget to clearly establish client and therapeutic goals. Are you clear on what concerns are motivating your clients to come to therapy? Do you understand where they feel the most pain, which is usually what motivates individuals to risk change? Have you clearly articulated to your clients what therapeutic goals you are striving to accomplish? Do they agree with these therapeutic goals as the focus of therapy? If clients express ambivalence or disagreement about your therapeutic goals, then you may need to reformulate your treatment plan.

Sometimes treatment can become stuck if the wrong modality is being used (e.g., individual versus couple or family). For example, a therapist may find that movement is slow when working primarily with a child. This may suggest that more work needs to be done with the family. With couples, it may be necessary to suggest one or both partners do some individual therapy before couple therapy can be optimally effective.

As you begin to intervene with your clients, ask yourself if they are responding well to the interventions you are using. One therapist began to realize that her client was not benefiting from an insight-oriented approach to therapy. Recognizing that this client was very concrete in her thinking, she began to incorporate more behavioral interventions, which were more successful in promoting change. It is also important to assess how receptive your clients are to direct suggestions. Some clients strongly resist being told what to do. One husband stated that he did not like being assigned homework because he hated being told to do it as a child. The therapist and couple agreed to call the assignments "relationship enhancement activities" to avoid this negative connotation. The therapist also emphasized that the activities were suggestions that the clients were free to do or not to do, and that they could have as much input as they wanted in designing them. This helped bypass the husband's resistance.

Finally, it is important to consider if you have overlooked some important barriers to change (see Chapter 3). Clients may have specific fears about change that need to be determined and overcome. You will need to help clients assess the extent to which these fears are realistic or not. Clients may also encounter unanticipated costs or consequences that hinder them from making the necessary changes. Family members may not like changes that a client is making, and put pressure on the individual to go back to his or her old pattern of doing things. Throughout the process, you need to consider possible negative consequences to change that your clients may face.

ASSESSING READINESS FOR TERMINATION

As clients make progress in therapy, the question of when to terminate becomes inevitable. In some cases, the client will be the first to raise the question. However, in more cases than not, it will be the therapist who will need to initiate the discussion. How will you know when it is time for termination?

There are a number of possible signs that your clients may be ready for termination. Obviously it should be considered once the client's goals have been met. This will be easier to evaluate if the goals have been clearly defined. Thus, how goals are set in the beginning may make it easier to determine when termination is appropriate. As clients become less distressed by their problems, they may start becoming less consistent in attending sessions. An increase in cancellations or no-shows may signal clients are ready to end therapy. Clients who are less distressed may also have less to talk about in therapy. They may engage in more social talk at the beginning of the session and take longer to transition to talking about their issues.

If you propose the idea of possible termination to your clients, it is important that you assess their reaction to termination. Some clients will express relief that the topic has been brought up, and will admit to having had similar thoughts. Other clients may be uncomfortable with the thought of ending therapy.

If clients seem uncomfortable with termination, it is important to determine why. Some clients will see the suggestion of termination as a sign of rejection, so you need to be attuned to any signals that your clients are interpreting your suggestion in this manner. Some clients can acknowledge that progress has been made but fear that the gains are fragile and will be lost if they discontinue therapy. In these situations, it may be prudent to consider spacing out therapy sessions to build confidence in their ability to maintain the gains they have made. Some clients, however, may feel that the suggestion to terminate is premature because they do not feel that they have accomplished as much as they need. It will be important to explore why there is a discrepancy between your perspective and those of your clients. Some clients will be extremely reluctant to end therapy because you are their primary source of social support. This may lead clients to overstate or even manufacture problems in order to maintain their relationship with you. This issue is best dealt with by anticipating it as a potential problem in the beginning of therapy. Clients with little or no social support are likely to have greater difficulty with termination (Patterson et al., 2009). If you recognize this risk early on, it may be feasible to expand their social support network to ease the pain of termination when it occurs.

CONCLUSION

Therapists often view assessment as something that is done at the beginning of therapy. However, as this chapter has illustrated, assessment is a process that never stops. Ongoing assessment is necessary to confirm our conceptualization of the case, and the effectiveness of our treatment interventions. It also helps us determine when clients have made sufficient progress to consider terminating therapy.

Summary of Assessment Tools, Instruments, and Mnemonics

ADULT ASSESSMENT

Assessment Tools

Listing and categorizing stressors (Chapter 5): control/no control; can be changed/no change possible; acute/chronic; normal/catastrophic; individual/family stressors

Kahneman Day Reconstruction Method for assessing well-being (Chapter 5)

Six rule-out rules (Chapter 6)

Mental status exam (Chapter 6)

Decision trees in DSM-IV-TR Appendix A (Chapter 6)

Screening questions for anxiety disorders (Chapter 6)

Structured Clinical Interview for DSM Disorders (SCID) (Chapter 6)

Assessment Instruments

Stress scales (Chapter 5): Perceived Stress Scale (PSS), Life Experience Survey (LES); Schedule of Recent Experiences

Happiness scales (Chapter 5): University of Pennsylvania scales, Positivity Self Test

Depression (Chapter 6): Beck Depression Inventory II (BDI-II); Center for Epidemiologic Studies Depression Scale (CES-D); Cornell Scale for Depression in Dementia; Geriatric Depression Scale; Hamilton Rating Scale for Depression; PHQ2 and PHQ9; Zung Self-Rating Depression Scale

Anxiety (Chapter 6): Beck Anxiety Inventory; Duke Anxiety–Depression Scale

(DUKE-AD); Hamilton Anxiety Scale (HAMA); Social Phobia Inventory
(SPIN)

General psychiatric measures (Chapter 6): Brief Symptom Inventory (BSI);
Mental Health Inventory (MHI); PRIME-MD–PHQ; SCL-90-R

Substance abuse (Chapter 6): Michigan Alcoholism Screening Test (MAST);
TWEAK

Mnemonics

ACTION for assessing harm to others (Chapter 4): Attitudes, Capacity, Thresholds crossed, Intent, Others' reactions and responses, Noncompliance

Depressed Patients Seem Anxious So Claim Psychiatrists for major categories
of disorders (Chapter 6): Depression and other mood disorders, Personality disorders, Substance abuse disorders, Anxiety disorders, Somatization
and eating disorders, Cognitive disorders, Psychotic disorders

SIGECAPS for neurovegetative symptoms of depression (Chapter 6): Sleep disorder, Interest deficit, Guilt, Energy deficit, Concentration deficit, Appetite disorder, Psychomotor retardation or agitation, Suicidality

IS PATH WARM for suicide risk factors (Chapter 6): Ideation, Substance abuse,
Purposelessness, Anxiety, Trapped, Hopelessness, Withdrawal, Anger,
Recklessness, Mood change

DIGFAST for symptoms of mania (Chapter 6): Distractibility, Indiscretion,
Grandiosity, Flight of ideas, Activity increase, Sleep deficit, Talkativeness

CAGE for alcohol abuse (Chapter 6): Cut down, Annoyed, Guilty, Eye opener

IDESPAIRR for borderline personality disorder (Chapter 6): Identity problem,
Disordered affect, Empty feeling, Suicidal behavior, Paranoia or dissociative symptoms, Abandonment terror, Impulsivity, Rage, Relationship
instability

CHILD AND ADOLESCENT ASSESSMENT

Assessment Tools

Play therapy (Chapter 7)

Nine general assessment questions (Chapter 8)

Biopsychosocial problem/strengths list (Chapter 8)

Assessment Instruments

Assessing child or adolescent behavior (Chapter 7): Achenbach System of Empirically Based Assessment; Behavior Assessment System for Children (BASC); Conners Comprehensive Behavior Rating Scales (CBRS); Personality Inventory for Children, 2nd edition (parent report); Student Behavior Survey (teacher report); Personality Inventory for Youth (self-report)

Mnemonics

JUST PEOPLE (Chapter 7): Judgment, Understanding others, Self-esteem, Temperament, Peers, Emotions, Outside interests, Psychopathology, Loved ones, Education

FAMILY ASSESSMENT

Assessment Tools

Genogram (Chapter 10)
Timeline (Chapter 10)
Sociogram (Chapter 10)

Assessment Instruments

Family functioning (Chapter 9): Family Adaptability and Cohesion Scales (FACES); Family Assessment Device (FAD); Family Assessment Measure (FAM); Family Environment Scale (FES)

Mnemonics

Four C's of parenting (Chapter 10): Consequences, Consistency, Calm, Charged batteries

COUPLE ASSESSMENT

Assessment Tools

Communication sample (Chapter 11)
Relationship history (Chapter 11)
Individual history for couple assessment (Chapter 11)
Sexual history (Chapter 12)

Assessment Instruments

Marital satisfaction or quality (Chapter 11): Dyadic Adjustment Scale (DAS); Revised Dyadic Adjustment Scale; Marital Adjustment Test (MAT); Marital Satisfaction Inventory

Marital stability (Chapter 11): Marital Status Inventory; Marital Instability Index

Relationship aggression (Chapter 11): Conflict Tactics Scale; Revised Conflict Tactics Scale

Personality (Chapter 11): Trait Descriptive Adjectives (TDA); Revised NEO Personality Inventory (NEO PI-R), Big Five Inventory (BFI); Myers–Briggs Type Indicator, Taylor–Johnson Temperament Analysis

Premarital inventories (Chapter 12): FOCCUS, PREPARE, RELATE

Mnemonics

Eight C's for assessing couple functioning (Chapter 11): Communication, Conflict resolution, Commitment, Contract, Caring/cohesion, Character, Culture, Children

Six A's for healing from infidelity (Chapter 12): Apology, Accept responsibility, Acknowledge how the person was hurt, Atonement, Answer why the affair happened, Accumulate trust

OTHER

Assessment Tools

Clinical interview, including open and closed questions (Chapter 2)
Assessment instruments (Chapter 2)
Behavioral observation (Chapter 2)
Physiological measures (Chapter 2)

Assessment Instruments

For measuring change (Chapter 13): BASIS-32; Brief Symptom Inventory; Outcome Questionnaire (OQ-45); Systemic Therapy Inventory of Change (STIC); Outcome Rating Scale (ORS); Session Rating Scale (SRS)

Mnemonics

RICE for administering instruments (Chapter 2): Rationale, Instructions, Confidentiality, Evaluate client response

References

Achenbach, T. M., & McConaughy, S. H. (2003). The Achenbach System of Empirically Based Assessment. In C. R. Reynolds & R. W. Kamphaus (Eds.), *Handbook of psychological and educational assessment of children* (2nd ed., pp. 406–430). New York: Guilford Press.

Alexopoulos, G. S., Abrams, R. C., Young, R. C., & Shamoian, C. A. (1988). Cornell Scale for Depression in Dementia. *Biological Psychiatry, 23*(3), 271–284.

Alonzo, D. J. (2005). Working with same-sex couples. In M. Harway (Ed.), *Handbook of couples therapy* (pp. 370–385). Hoboken, NJ: Wiley.

American Psychiatric Association. (2000). *Diagnostic and statistical manual of mental disorders* (4th ed., text rev.). Washington, DC: Author.

Anderson, C. (2003). The diversity, strength, and challenges of single-parent households. In F. Walsh (Ed.), *Normal family processes* (3rd ed., pp. 121–152). New York: Guilford Press.

Anxiety Disorders Association of America. (2009). Retrieved July 10, 2009, from *www.adaa.org.*

Ariel, J., & McPherson, D. W. (2000). Therapy with lesbian and gay parents and their children. *Journal of Marital and Family Therapy, 26,* 421–432.

Attarian, H. P. (2000). Helping patients who say they cannot sleep. *Postgraduate Medicine, 107*(3), 127–140.

Barkley, R. (2005). *ADHD and the nature of self-control.* New York: Guilford Press.

Basson, R. (2007). Sexual desire/arousal disorders in women. In S. R. Leiblum (Ed.), *Principles and practice of sex therapy* (4th ed., pp. 25–53). New York: Guilford Press.

Beach, S. (2003). Affective disorders. *Journal of Marital and Family Therapy, 29,* 247–261.

Beach, S., Wamboldt, M., Kaslow, N., Heyman, R., First, M., Underwood, L., et al. (2006). *Relational process and DSM-V.* Washington DC: American Psychiatric Publishing.

Beach, S., Wamboldt, M., Kaslow, N., Heyman, R., & Reiss, D. (2006). Describing relationship problems in DSM-V: Toward better guidance for research and clinical practice. *Journal of Family Psychology, 20,* 359–368.

Beck, A. T., Epstein, N., Brown, G., & Steer, R. A. (1988). An inventory for measuring clinical anxiety: Psychometric properties. *Journal of Consulting and Clinical Psychology, 56,* 893–897.

Beck, A. T., Steer, R. A., & Brown, G. K. (1996). *Manual for the Beck Depression Inventory–II.* San Antonio, TX: Pearson.

Becker, D., & Liddle, H. A. (2001). Family therapy with unmarried African American mothers and their adolescents. *Family Process, 40,* 413–427.

Belfort, M. (2007, October 30). Emotional abyss; Physical cause? *New York Times,* pp. F5.

Belsky, J., & Kelly, J. (1994). *The transition to parenthood: How a first child changes a marriage and why some couples grow closer and others apart.* New York: Dell.

Ben-Shahar, T. (2007). *Happier: Learn the secrets to daily joy and lasting fulfillment.* New York: McGraw-Hill.

Birchler, G. R. (1983). Marital dysfunction. In M. Hersen (Ed.), *Outpatient behavioral therapy: A clinical guide* (pp. 229–269). New York: Grune & Stratton.

Birchler, G. R., Doumas, D. M., & Fals-Stewart, W. S. (1999). The seven Cs: A behavioral systems framework for evaluating marital distress. *The Family Journal: Counseling and Therapy for Couples and Families, 7,* 253–264.

Bograd, M., & Mederos, F. (1999). Battering and couples therapy: Universal screening and selection of treatment modality. *Journal of Marital and Family Therapy, 25,* 291–312.

Booth, A., & Edwards, J. (1983). Measuring marital instability. *Journal of Marriage and the Family, 45,* 387–394.

Borum, B., & Reddy, M. (2001). Assessing violence risk in Tarasoff situations: A fact-based model of inquiry. *Behavioral Sciences and the Law, 19,* 375–385.

Boss, P. (1998). *Ambiguous loss.* Cambridge, MA: Harvard University Press.

Bowen, M. (1991). Family reaction to death. In F. Walsh & M. McGoldrick (Eds.), *Living beyond loss: Death in the family* (pp. 79–92). New York: Norton.

Bowlby, J. (1980). *Attachment and loss* (Vol. III). New York: Basic Books.

Braaten, E., & Felopulos, G. (2004). *Straight talk about psychological testing for kids.* New York: Guilford Press.

Bradburn, N., Sudman, S., & Wansink, B. (2004). *Asking questions: The definitive guide to questionnaire design—For market research, political polls, and social and health questionnaires.* San Francisco: Wiley.

Bray, J. H. (2008). Couple therapy with remarried partners. In A. S. Gurman (Ed.), *Clinical handbook of couple therapy* (4th ed., pp. 499–519). New York: Guilford Press.

Buck, J. N. (1977). *House–Tree–Person projective drawing technique: Revised manual and interpretative guide.* Los Angeles: Western Psychological Services.

Burlingame, G.M., Wells, M.G., Lambert, M.J., Cox, J., Latkowski, M., & Justice, D. (2005). *Administration and scoring manual for the Youth Outcome Questionnaire (Y-OQ.2.2).* Salt Lake City, UT: American Professional Credentialing Services.

Burns, R. C., & Kaufman, S. H. (1972). *Actions, styles and symbols in Kinetic Family Drawings (K-F-D): An interpretative manual.* New York: Brunner-Routledge.

Busby, D. M., Christensen, C., Crane, D. R., & Larson, J. H. (1995). A revision of the Dyadic Adjustment Scale for use with distressed and nondistressed couples: Construct hierarchy and multidimensional scales. *Journal of Marital and Family Therapy, 21,* 289–308.

Carey, B. (2008, December 17). Psychiatrists revise the book of human troubles. *New York Times,* p. 18.

Carlat, D. (1998). The psychiatric review of symptoms: A screening tool for family physicians. *American Family Physician, 58,* 1617–1624.

Carter, B., & McGoldrick, M. (2005). *The expanded family life cycle: Individual, family, and social perspectives.* New York: Allyn & Bacon.

Christakis, N., & Fowler, J. (2007). The spread of obesity in a large social network over 32 years. *New England Journal of Medicine, 357,* 370–379.

Christakis, N., & Fowler, J. (2009). *Connected: The surprising power of our social networks and how they shape our lives.* New York: Little, Brown.

Clarke-Stewart, A. (2006). *Divorce: Causes and consequences.* New Haven, CT: Yale University Press.

Cohen, S. (2004). Social relationships and health. *American Psychologist, 59,* 676–685.

Cohen, S., Kamarck, T., & Mermelstein, R. (1983). A global measure of perceived stress. *Journal of Health and Social Behavior, 24,* 386–396.

Combrinck-Graham, L. (1985). A developmental model for family systems. *Family Process, 24,* 139–150.

Conners, C. K. (2008). *Conners Comprehensive Child Behavior Rating Scales manual.* North Tonawanda, NY: MHS.

Conners, C. K. (2009). *Conners Early Childhood manual.* North Tonawanda, NY: MHS.

Connor, K. M., Davidson, J. R. T., Churchill, L. E., Sherwood, A., Foa, E., & Weisler, R. H. (2000). Psychometric properties of the Social Phobia Inventory (SPIN): New self-rating scale. *British Journal of Psychiatry, 176,* 379–386.

Costa, P. T., & McCrae, R. R. (1992). *NEO PI-R Professional Manual.* Odessa, FL: Psychological Assessment Resources.

Cowan, C. P., & Cowan, P. A. (2000). *When partners become parents.* New York: Basic Books.

Crane, D. R., Allgood, S. M., Larson, J. H., & Griffin, W. (1990). Assessing marital quality with distressed and nondistressed couples: A comparison and equivalency table for three frequently used measures. *Journal of Marriage and the Family, 52,* 87–93.

Csikszentmihalyi, M. (1998). *Finding flow: The psychology of engagement with everyday life.* New York: Basic Books.

Derogatis, L. R. (1993). *Brief Symptom Inventory: Administration, scoring, and procedures manual* (3rd ed.). Minneapolis, MN: National Computer Systems.

de Shazer, S. (1988). *Clues: Investigating solutions in brief therapy.* New York: Norton.

Diener, E., & Biswas-Diener, R. (2008). *Happiness: Unlocking the mysteries of psychological wealth.* Malden, MA: Blackwell.

Duncan, B. L., Miller, S. D., Sparks, J. A., Claud, D. A., Reynolds, L. R., Brown, J., et al. (2003). The Session Rating Scale: Preliminary psychometric properties of a "working" alliance measure. *Journal of Brief Therapy, 3*(1), 3–12.

Duncan, B. L., Sparks, J. A., Miller, S. D., Bohanske, R. T., & Claud, D. A. (2006). Giving youth a voice: A preliminary study of the reliability and validity of a brief outcome measure for children, adolescents, and caretakers. *Journal of Brief Therapy, 5*(2), 71–87.

Edwards, D. L., & Gil, E. (1986). *Breaking the cycle: Assessment and treatment of child abuse and neglect.* Los Angeles: Association for Advanced Training in the Behavioral Sciences.

Edwards, T. M. (2002). A place at the table: Integrating diet and nutrition into family therapy practice. *American Journal of Family Therapy, 30,* 243–255.

Eisen, S. V., Grob, M. C., & Klein, A. A. (1986). BASIS: The development of a self-report measure for psychiatric inpatient evaluation. *Psychiatric Hospital, 17,* 166–171.

Emmons, R., & McCullough, M. (2004). *The psychology of gratitude.* New York: Oxford University Press.

Engel, G. L. (1977). The need for a new medical model: A challenge for biomedicine. *Science, 196,* 129–136.

Epstein, N. B., Baldwin, L. M., & Bishop, D. S. (1983). The McMaster Family Assessment Device. *Journal of Marital and Family Therapy, 9,* 171–180.

Epstein, R. M., & Borrell-Carrio, F. (2005). The biopsychosocial model: Exploring six impossible things. *Families, Systems, & Health, 23,* 426–431.

Ewing J. A. (1984). Detecting alcoholism: The CAGE questionnaire. *Journal of the American Medical Association, 252,* 1905–1907.

Falicov, C. J. (2002). Ambiguous loss: Risk and resilience in Latino families. In M. Suarez-Orozco & M. Paez (Eds.), *Latinos: Remaking American* (pp. 274–288). Berkeley: University of California Press.

Falicov, C. J. (2007). Working with transnational immigrants: Expanding meanings of family, community, and culture. *Family Process, 46,* 157–171.

Faraone, S. (2003). *Straight talk about your child's mental health.* New York: Guilford Press.

Fischer, J., & Corcoran, K. (2007). *Measures for clinical practice: A sourcebook: Vol. 1. Couples, families, and children* (4th ed.). New York: Oxford University Press.

Frances, A., & First, M. (1995). Assessment, diagnosis and treatment planning. Workshop syllabus, Institute for Behavioral Healthcare, Los Angeles, CA.

Fredman, N., & Sherman, R. (1987). *Handbook of measurements for marriage and family therapy.* Philadelphia: Brunner/Mazel.

Fredrickson, B. L. (2009). *Positivity: Groundbreaking research reveals how to embrace the hidden strength of positive emotions, overcome negativity, and thrive.* New York: Crown.

Friedman, H., Rohrbaugh, M., & Krakauer, S. (1988). The time-line genogram: Highlighting temporal aspects of family relationships. *Family Process, 27,* 293–303.

Ganong, L., Coleman, M., Fine, M., & Martin, P. (1999). Stepparents' affinity-seeking and affinity–maintaining strategies with stepchildren. *Journal of Family Issues, 20,* 299–327.

Gil, E. (2006). *Helping abused and traumatized children.* New York: Guilford Press.

Goldberg, L. R. (1992). The development of markers for the Big-Five factor structure. *Psychological Assessment, 4,* 26–42.

Gottman, J. (1994). *What predicts divorce?: The relationship between marital process and marital outcomes.* Hillsdale, NJ: Erlbaum.

Gottman, J. M. (1999). *The marriage clinic: A scientifically based marital therapy.* New York: Norton.

Gottman, J. M., DeClaire, J., & Siegel, D. (1997). *The heart of parenting: Raising an emotionally intelligent child.* New York: Simon & Schuster.

Green, R.-J., & Mitchell, V. (2008). Gay and lesbian couples in therapy: Minority stress, relational ambiguity, and families of choice. In A. S. Gurman (Ed.), *Clinical handbook of couple therapy* (4th ed., pp. 662–680). New York: Guilford Press.

Greene, K., & Bogo, M. (2002). The different faces of intimate violence: Implications for assessment and treatment. *Journal of Marital and Family Therapy, 28,* 455–466.

Grotevant, H. D., & Carlson, C. I. (1989). *Family assessment: A guide to methods and measures.* New York: Guilford Press.

Guerin, P. J., Fogarty, T. F., Fay, L. F., & Kautto, J. G. (1996). *Working with relationship triangles: One-two-three of psychotherapy.* New York: Guilford Press.

Hamilton, M. (1959). The assessment of anxiety stated by rating. *British Journal of Psychology, 32,* 52–55.

Hamilton, M. (1960). A rating scale for depression. *Journal of Neurology, Neurosurgery, and Psychiatry, 23,* 56–62.

Hampson, R. B., & Beavers, W. R. (2007). Observational assessment of couples and families. In L. Sperry (Ed.), *Assessment of couples and families: Con-*

temporary and cutting-edge strategies (pp. 91–115). New York: Brunner-Routledge.

Harris, R. (2009). *ACT with love: Stop struggling, reconcile differences, and strengthen your relationship with acceptance and commitment therapy.* Oakland, CA: New Harbinger.

Hartmann, U., & Waldinger, M. D. (2007). Treatment of delayed ejaculation. In S. R. Leiblum (Ed.), *Principles and practice of sex therapy* (4th ed., pp. 241–276). New York: Guilford Press.

Hetherington, E.M., & Stanley-Hagan, M. (2002). Parenting in divorced and remarried families. In M. Bornstein (Ed.), *Handbook of parenting* (2nd ed., pp. 287–316). Mahwah, NJ: Erlbaum.

Hiebert, W. J., Gillespie, J. P., & Stahmann, R. F. (1993). *Dynamic assessment in couple therapy.* New York: Lexington Books.

Hirshfeld-Becker, D., & Geller, D. (2006, March). *Anxiety disorders in childhood and adolescence.* Presentation at the Child and Adolescent Psychopharmacology Conference, Boston, MA.

Holmes, T. H., & Rahe, R. H. (1967). Holmes–Rahe life changes scale. *Journal of Psychosomatic Research, 11,* 213–218.

Holtzworth-Munroe, A., Clements, K., & Farris, C. (2005). Working with couples who have experienced physical aggression. In M. Harway (Ed.), *Handbook of couples therapy* (pp. 289–312). Hoboken, NJ: Wiley.

Hooley, J. M. (2007). Expressed emotion and relapse of psychopathology. *Annual Review of Clinical Psychology, 3,* 329–352.

Horwitz, S. H. (1997). Treating families with traumatic loss: Transitional family therapy. In C. Figley, B. Bride, & N. Mazza (Eds.), *Death and trauma: The traumatology of grieving* (pp. 211–230). London: Taylor & Francis.

Horwitz, M. J., Siegel, B., Holen, A., Bonanno, G. A., Milbrath, C., & Stinson, C. H. (1997). Diagnostic criteria for complicated grief disorder. *American Journal of Psychiatry, 154,* 904–910.

Jacobson, N. S., & Truax, P. (1991). Clinical significance: A statistical approach to defining meaningful change in psychotherapy research. *Journal of Consulting and Clinical Psychology, 59,* 12–19.

John, O. P., Donahue, E. M., & Kentle, R. L. (1991). *The Big Five Inventory—Versions 4a and 54.* Berkeley: University of California, Berkeley, Institute of Personality and Social Research.

John, O. P., & Srivastava, S. (1999). The Big-Five trait taxonomy: History, measurement, and theoretical perspectives. In L. A. Pervin & O. P. John (Eds.), *Handbook of personality: Theory and research* (Vol. 2, pp. 102–138). New York: Guilford Press.

Johnson, S. M., Makinen, M., & Millikin, J. (2001). Attachment injuries in couple relationships: A new perspective on impasses in couple therapy. *Journal of Marital and Family Therapy, 27,* 145–155.

Kahneman, D., & Krueger, A. (2004). A survey method for characterizing daily life experience: The Day Reconstruction Method. *Science, 306,* 1776–1780.

Kamarck, T., & Anderson, B. (2006, June). *Assessment of psychological stress.* Presentation at the Pittsburgh Mind–Body Center Summer Institute, Pittsburgh, PA.

Keirsey, D. (1998). *Please understand me II: Temperament, character, intelligence.* Del Mar, CA: Prometheus Nemesis.

Keltner, D. (2009). *Born to be good.* New York: Norton.

Kerr, M. E., & Bowen, M. (1988). *Family evaluation.* New York: Norton.

Kessler, R., Adler, L., Ames, M., Demler, O., Faraone, S., Hiripi, E., et al. (2005). The World Health Organization Adult ADHD Self-Report Scale (ASRS): A short screening scale for use in the general population. *Psychological medicine, 35,* 245–256.

Kessler, R., Adler, L., Barkley, R., Biderman, J., Conners, C., Demler, O., et al. (2006). The prevalence and correlates of adult ADHD in the United States: Results from the National Comorbidity Survey Replication. *American Journal of Psychiatry, 163,* 716–723.

Kessler, R., Berglund, P., Demler, O., Jin, R., & Walters, E. (2005). Lifetime prevalence and age-of-onset distribution of DSM-IV disorders in the National Comorbidity Survey Replication. *Archives of General Psychiatry, 6,* 593–602.

Kessler, R., Chiu, W., Demler, O., & Walters, E. (2005). Prevalence, severity, and comorbidity of 12-month DSM-IV disorders in the National Comorbidity Survey Replication. *Archives of General Psychiatry, 62,* 617–627.

Ketring, S. A. (2007, September/October). Child physical abuse and neglect. *Family Therapy Magazine,* 40–49.

Kiecolt-Glaser, J., & Newton, T. (2001). Marriage and health: His and hers. *Psychological Bulletin, 127*(4), 472–503.

Kornfield, J. (2009). *The wise heart.* New York: Bantam Press.

Kroeger, O., & Thuesen, J. M. (1988). *Type talk: The 16 personality types that determine how we live, love, and work.* New York: Dell.

L'Abate, L., & Bagarozzi, D. A. (1993). *Sourcebook for marriage and family evaluation.* New York: Brunner/Mazel.

Lachar, D., & Gruber, C. P. (2003). Multisource and multidimensional objective assessment of adjustment: The Personality Inventory for Children, second edition; Personality Inventory for Youth; and Student Behavior Survey. In C. R. Reynolds & R. W. Kamphaus (Eds.), *Handbook of psychological and educational assessment of children* (2nd ed., pp. 337–367). New York: Guilford Press.

Lambert, M. J., & Hawkins, E. J. (2004). Measuring outcome in professional practice: Considerations in selecting and using brief outcome instruments. *Professional Psychology: Research and Practice, 35,* 492–499.

Lambert, M.J., Morton, J. J., Hatfield, D., Harmon, C., Hamilton, S., Reid, R. C., et al. (2004). *Administration and Scoring Manual for the OQ-45.2.* Orem, UT: American Professional Credentialing Services.

Larson, J. H., Newell, K., Topham, G., & Nichols, S. (2002). A review of three comprehensive premarital assessment questionnaires. *Journal of Marital and Family Therapy, 28,* 233–239.

Leiblum, S. R. (Ed.). (2007). *Principles and practice of sex therapy* (4th ed.). New York: Guilford Press.

LeMasters, E. E. (1957). Parenthood as crises. *Marriage and Family Living, 19,* 352–355.

Levine, M. (2002). A *mind at a time*. New York: Simon & Schuster.

Levine, M. (2003). *The myth of laziness*. New York: Simon & Schuster.

Lindblad-Goldberg, M. (1989). Successful minority single-parent families. In L. Combrinck-Graham (Ed.), *Children in family contexts* (pp. 116–134). New York: Guilford Press.

Locke, H., & Wallace, K. (1959). Short marital adjustment and prediction tests: Their reliability and validity. *Marriage and Family Living, 21,* 251–255.

Lucht, M., Jahn, U., Barnow, S., & Freyberger, H. J. (2002). The use of a symptom checklist (SCL-90-R) as an easy method to estimate the relapse risk after alcoholism detoxification. *European Addiction Research, 8,* 190–194.

Mash, E., & Barkley, R. (Eds.). (2007). *Assessment of childhood disorders* (4th ed.). New York: Guilford Press.

McCrae, R. R., & Costa, P. T. (1989). Reinterpreting the Myers–Briggs Type Indicator from the perspective of the Five-Factor model of personality. *Journal of Personality, 57,* 17–40.

McCubbin, H. I., Thompson, A. I., & McCubbin, M. A. (1996). *Family assessment: Resiliency, coping, and adaptation—Inventories for research and practice*. Madison: University of Wisconsin.

McGoldrick, M., & Carter, B. (2003). The family life cycle. In F. Walsh (Ed.), *Normal family processes* (3rd ed., pp. 375–398). New York: Guilford Press.

McGoldrick, M., Gerson, R., & Petry, S. (2008). *Genograms: Assessment and intervention* (3rd ed.). New York: Norton.

Milkowitz, D. (2008). *Bipolar disorder: A family-focused treatment approach* (2nd ed.). New York: Guilford Press.

Miller, S. D., Duncan, B. L., Brown, J., Sorrell, R., & Chalk, M. B. (2006). Using formal client feedback to improve retention and outcome: Making ongoing, real-time assessment feasible. *Journal of Brief Therapy, 5*(1), 5–22.

Miller, S. D., Duncan, B. L., Brown, J., Sparks, J. A., & Claud, D. A. (2003). The Outcome Rating Scale: A preliminary study of the reliability, validity, and feasibility of a brief visual analog measure. *Journal of Brief Therapy, 2*(2), 91–100.

Miller, W. R., & Rollnick, S. (2002). *Motivational interviewing: Lessons preparing people for change* (2nd ed.). New York: Guilford Press.

Moos, R. H., & Moos, B. S. (1986). *Family Environment Scale manual* (Rev. ed.). Palo Alto, CA: Consulting Psychologists Press.

Morrison, J. (2007). *Diagnosis made easier*. New York: Guilford Press.

Myers, D. (2000). The funds, friends, and faith of happy people. *American Psychologist, 55*(1), 56–67.

Myers, D. (2008). Religion and human flourishing. In M. Eid & R. Larsen (Eds.), *The science of subjective well-being* (pp. 323–346). New York: Guilford Press.

Myers, I. B., McCaulley, M. H., Quenk, N. L., & Hammer, A. L. (1998). *MBTI Manual: A guide to the development and use of the Myers–Briggs Type Indicator instrument* (3rd ed.). Mountain View, CA: CPP.

Napier, A. Y., & Whitaker, C. (1973). Problems of the beginning family therapist. *Seminars in Psychiatry, 5,* 229–241.

National Center for Injury Prevention and Control. (2003). *Costs of intimate partner violence against women in the United States.* Atlanta, GA: Centers for Disease Control and Prevention.

Nichols, M. P., & Schwartz, R. C. (2007). *Family therapy: Concepts & methods* (8th ed.). New York: Allyn & Bacon.

Nichols, W. C. (1996). *Treating people in families: An integrative framework.* New York: Guilford Press.

Nichols, W. C., & Everett, C. A. (1986). *Systemic family therapy.* New York: Guilford Press.

Nichols, W. C., & Pace-Nichols, M. A. (2000). Family development and family therapy. In W. C. Nichols, M. A. Pace-Nichols, D. S. Becvar, & A. Y. Napier (Eds.), *Handbook of family development and intervention* (pp. 3–22). New York: Wiley.

Nock, M., & Kessler, R. (2006). Prevalence of and risk factors for suicide attempts versus suicide gestures: Analysis of the national comorbidity survey. *Journal of Abnormal Psychology, 115,* 616–623.

Noller, P., Feeney, J. A., Bonnell, D., & Callan, V. J. (1994). A longitudinal study of conflict in early marriage. *Journal of Social and Personal Relationships, 11,* 233–252.

Olson, D.H., & Gorall, D.M. (2003). Circumplex model of marital and family systems. In F. Walsh (Ed.), *Normal family processes* (3rd ed., pp. 514–547). New York: Guilford Press.

Olson, D. H., Gorall, D. M., & Tiesel, J. W. (2007). FACES IV and the circumplex model: Validation study. *Journal of Family Therapy, 22,* 144–167.

Olson, D. H., Russell, C. S., & Sprenkle, D. H. (1989). *Circumplex model: Systemic assessment and treatment of families.* New York: Haworth Press.

Papernow, P. L. (1993). *Becoming a stepfamily.* San Francisco: Jossey-Bass.

Parkerson, G. R., Jr., & Broadhead, W.E. (1997). Screening for anxiety and depression in primary care with the Duke Anxiety-Depression Scale (DUKE-AD). *Family Medicine, 29*(3), 177–181.

Parkes, C. M. (1972). *Bereavement: Studies of grief in adult life.* New York: International Universities Press.

Patterson, J., Albala, A., McCahill, M., & Edwards, T. (2006). *The therapist's guide to psychopharmacology: Working with patients, families, and physicians to optimize care.* New York: Guilford Press.

Patterson, J., Williams, L., Edwards, T., Chamow, L., & Grauf-Grounds, C. (2009). *Essential skills in family therapy: From the first interview to termination* (2nd ed.). New York: Guilford Press.

Patterson, T. (1999). *The couple and family clinical documentation sourcebook: A comprehensive collection of mental health practice forms, inventories, handouts, and records.* New York: Wiley.

Pendegast, E., & Sherman, C. O. (1977), A guide to the genogram. *Family, 5,* 3–13.

Pinsof, W. M., & Chambers, A.L. (2009). Empirically informed systemic psychotherapy: Tracking client change and therapist behavior during therapy. In J. Bray & M. Stanton (Eds.), *The Wiley–Blackwell Handbook of Family Psychology* (pp. 431–446). Oxford, UK: Blackwell.

Prochaska, J. O., Norcross, J. C., & DiClemente, C. C. (1995). *Changing for good: A revolutionary six-stage program for overcoming bad habits and moving your life positively forward.* New York: Avon.

Qualls, S. H. (2000). Therapy with aging families: Rationale, opportunities, and challenges. *Aging & Mental Health, 4,* 191–199.

Radloff, L. S. (1977). The CES-D scale: A self-report depression scale for research in the general population. *Applied Psychological Measurement, 1,* 385–401.

Rahimian, J., Bergman, J., Brown, G., & Ceniceros, S. (2006). Human sexuality. In D. Wedding & M. Stuber (Eds.), *Behavior and medicine* (4th ed., pp. 153–164). Cambridge, MA: Hogrefe Press.

Rapee, R., Wignall, D., Spence, S., Cobham, V., & Lyneham, H. (2008). *Helping your anxious child* (2nd Ed). Oakland, CA: New Harbinger.

Regier, D. A., Boyd, J. H., Burke, J. D., & Rae, D. A. (1988). One-month prevalence of mental disorders in the United States. *Archives of General Psychiatry, 45,* 977–986.

Riggs, D. S., Caulfield, M. B., & Street, A. E. (2000). Risk for domestic violence: Factors associated with perpetration and victimization. *Journal of Clinical Psychology, 56,* 1289–1316.

Roan, S. (2010, February 10). Revising the book on mental illness. *Los Angeles Times.* Retrieved May 19, 2010, from *www.latimes.com/news/science/la-sci-dsm10-2010feb10,0,3283581.story?track=rss.*

Rolland, J. S. (1994). *Families, illness, and disability.* New York: Basic Books.

Rolland, J. S. (1998). Beliefs and collaboration in illness: Evolution over time. *Families, Systems, and Health, 16,* 7–25.

Ruddy, N. B., & McDaniel, S. H. (2008). Couple therapy and medical issues: Working with couples facing illness. In A. S. Gurman (Ed.), *Clinical handbook of couple therapy* (4th ed., pp. 618–640). New York: Guilford Press.

Russell, M. (1994). New assessment tools for drinking in pregnancy: T-ACE, TWEAK, and others. *Alcohol Health and Research World, 18*(1), 55–61.

Sapolsky, R. (1998). *Why zebras don't get ulcers: An updated guide to stress, stress related diseases, and coping* (2nd ed.). New York: Henry Holt.

Sarason, I., Johnson, J., & Siegel, J. (1978). Assessing the impact of life changes: Development of the life experiences survey. *Journal of Consulting and Clinical Psychology, 46*(5), 932–946.

Schacht, R. L., Dimidjian, S., George, W. H., & Berns, S. B. (2009). Domestic violence assessment procedures among couple therapists. *Journal of Marital and Family Therapy, 35,* 47–59.

Sedlack, A., & Broadhurst, D. (1996). *Third national incidence study of child abuse and neglect: Final report.* Washington, DC: U.S. Department of Health and Human Services.

Selzer, M. (1971). The Michigan Alcoholism Screening Test (MAST): The quest for a new diagnostic instrument. *American Journal of Psychiatry, 127,* 1653–1658.

Shapiro, A. F., & Gottman, J. M. (2005). Effects on marriage of a psycho-communicative-educational intervention with couples undergoing the transition to parenthood, evaluation at 1-year post intervention. *Journal of Family Communication, 5,* 1–24.

Shapiro, A. F., Gottman, J. M., & Carrere, S. (2000). The baby and the marriage: Identifying factors that buffer against decline in marital satisfaction after the first baby arrives. *Journal of Family Psychology, 14,* 345–360.

Shea, S. C. (1999). *The practical art of suicide assessment.* New York: Wiley.

Shear, K., Frank, E., Houck, P. R., & Reynolds, C. F. (2005). Treatment of complicated grief: A randomized controlled trial. *Journal of the American Medical Association, 293,* 2601–2608.

Shenk, J. (2009). What makes us happy? *The Atlantic.* Retrieved May 20, 2009, from *http://theatlantic.com/doc/200906/happiness.*

Shields, C. G., King, D. A., & Wynne, L. C. (1995). Interventions with later life families. In R. H. Mikesell, D. Lusterman, & S. H. McDaniel (Eds.), *Integrating family therapy: Handbook of family psychology and systems theory* (pp. 141–158). Washington, DC: American Psychological Association.

Siegel, D. (1999). *The developing mind.* New York: Guilford Press.

Simmons, T., & O'Neill, G. (2001, September). *Households and Families: 2000–Census Brief.* Retrieved August 26, 2010, from *http://www.census.gov/prod/2001pubs/c2kbr01-8.pdf.*

Skinner, H. A., Steinhauer, P. D., & Santa-Barbera, J. (1984). *The Family Assessment Measure: Administration and interpretation guide.* Toronto: Multi-Health Systems. (Available from Addiction Research Foundation, Toronto)

Skoog, I., Nilsson, L., Palmertz, B. Andreasson, L., & Svanborg, A. (1993). A population-based study of dementia in 85-year-olds. *New England Journal of Medicine, 328,* 153–158.

Snyder, D. K. (1997). *Manual for the Marital Satisfaction Inventory—Revised.* Los Angeles: Western Psychological Services.

Spanier, G. B. (1976). Measuring dyadic adjustment: New scales for assessing the quality of marriage and similar dyads. *Journal of Marriage and the Family, 38,* 15–28.

Spencer, T. (2006, March). *Juvenile Depression.* Presentation at the Child and Adolescent Psychopharmacology Conference, Boston, MA.

Sperry, L. (Ed.). (2004). *Assessment of couples and families: Contemporary and cutting-edge strategies.* New York: Brunner-Routledge.

Spitzer, R., Kroenke, K., & Williams, J. (1999). Validation and utility of a self-report version of PRIME-MD: The PHQ Primary Care Study. *Journal of the American Medical Association, 282,* 1737–1744.

Spitzer, R. L., Williams, J. B., Gibbon M., & First, M. B. (1992). The Structured Clinical Interview for DSM-III-R (SCID-I): History, rationale, and description. *Archives of General Psychiatry, 49*(8), 624–629.

Spitzer, R., Williams, J., Kroenke, K., Linzer, M., & Verloin deGruy, F. (1994). Utility of new procedure for diagnosing mental disorders in primary-care: The PRIME-MD 1000 study. *Journal of the American Medical Association, 272,* 1749–56.

Stahmann, R. F., & Hiebert, W. J. (1997). *Premarital and remarital counseling: The professional's handbook.* San Francisco: Jossey-Bass.

Stanley, S. M., Rhoades, G. K., & Markman, H. J. (2006). Sliding versus deciding: Inertia and the premarital cohabitation effect. *Family Relations, 55,* 499–509.

Stanton, M. D. (1992). The time line and the "why now"? question: A technique and rationale for therapy, training, organizational consultation and research. *Journal of Marital and Family Therapy, 18,* 331–343.

Stith, S. M., Rosen, K. H., & McCollum, E. E. (2003). Effectiveness of couples treatment for spouse abuse. *Journal of Marital and Family Therapy, 29,* 407–426.

Straus, M. A. (1979). Measuring intrafamily conflict and violence: The Conflict Tactics Scale. *Journal of Marriage and Family, 41,* 75–88.

Straus, M. A., Hamby, S. L., Boney-McCoy, S., & Sugarman, D. B. (1996). The Revised Conflict Tactics Scale (CTS2): Development and preliminary psychometric data. *Journal of Family Issues, 17,* 283–316.

Tannen, D. (1990). *You just don't understand: Women and men in conversation.* New York: William Morrow.

Taylor, R. M., & Morrison, L. P. (2007). *Taylor–Johnson Temperament Analysis manual.* Thousand Oaks, CA: Psychological Publications.

Terling-Watt, T. (2001). Explaining divorce: An examination of the relationship between marital charactistics and divorce. *Journal of Divorce and Remarriage, 35,* 125–145.

Thorpe, J., Kamphaus, R. W., & Reynolds, C. R. (2003). The Behavior Assessment System for Children. In C. R. Reynolds & R. W. Kamphaus (Eds.), *Handbook of psychological and educational assessment of children* (2nd ed., pp. 387–405). New York: Guilford Press.

Touliatos, J., Perlmutter, B. F., & Straus, M. A. (Eds.). (2001). *Handbook of family measurement techniques* (Vols. 1–3). Thousand Oaks, CA: Sage.

Turecki, S., & Tonner, L. (2000). *The difficult child* (2nd ed.). New York: Bantam Books.

Veit, C., & Ware, J. (1983). The structure of psychological distress and well-being in general populations. *Journal of Consulting and Clinical Psychology, 51,* 730–742.

Visher, E. B., & Visher, J. S. (1988). *Old loyalties, new ties: Therapeutic strategies with stepfamilies.* New York: Brunner/Mazel.

Waite, L., & Hughes, M. (2009). Marital biography and health midlife. *Journal of Health and Social Behavior, 50*, 344–359.

Walsh, F. (2006). *Strengthening family resilience* (2nd ed.). New York: Guilford Press.

Walsh, F. (Ed.). (2009). *Spiritual resources in family therapy* (2nd ed.). New York: Guilford Press.

Weber, T., & Levine, F. (1995). Engaging the family: An integrative approach. In R. H. Mikesell, D. Lusterman, & S. H. McDaniel (Eds.), *Integrating family therapy: Handbook of family psychology and systems theory* (pp. 45–72). Washington, DC: American Psychological Association.

Weiss, R., & Cerrato, M. (1980). The marital status inventory: Development of a measure of dissolution potential. *American Journal of Family Therapy, 8*, 80–85.

Whitaker, C., & Napier, A. Y. (1978). *The family crucible*. New York: Harper & Row.

Whiting, J. B., & Crane, D. R. (2003). Distress and divorce: Establishing cutoff scores for the Marital Status Inventory. *American Journal of Family Therapy, 25*, 195–205.

Williams, L. (2007). Premarital counseling. In J. L. Wetchler (Ed.), *Handbook of clinical issues in couple therapy* (pp. 207–217). Binghamton, NY: Haworth Press.

Williams, L. M., & Cushing, E. (2005). The four C's of parenting. In K. M. Hertlein & D. Viers (Eds.), *The couple and family therapist's notebook: Homework, handouts, and activities for use in psychotherapy* (pp. 65–69). New York: Haworth Press.

Williams, L. M., & Lawler, M. G. (1998). Interchurch couples: The issue of acceptance. *Pastoral Psychology, 47*(1), 33–47.

Williams, P., & Thayer, J. (2009). Executive functioning and health: Introduction to the special series. *Annals of Behavioral Medicine, 37*, 101–105.

Wolff, D. (1999). *Child abuse: Implications for child development and psychopathology,* (2nd ed., Vol. 10). Thousand Oaks, CA: Sage.

World Health Organization. (2009). *Suicide Prevention (SUPRE)*. Retrieved March 26, 2009, from *www.who.int/mental_health/prevention/suicide/suicideprevent/en/index.html*.

World Health Organization. (2000). *Preventing suicide: A resource for general physicians*. Retrieved March 26, 2009, from *www.who.int/mental_health/media/en/56.pdf*.

Wozniak, J. (2006, March). *Juvenile mania*. Presentation at the Child and Adolescent Psychopharmacology Conference, Boston, MA.

Yesavage, J. A., Brink, T. L., Rose, T. L., Lum, O., Huang, V., Adey, M. B., et al. (1983). Development and validation of a geriatric depression screening scale: A preliminary report. *Journal of Psychiatric Research, 17*, 37–49.

Zung, W. W. (1965). A self-rating depression scale. *Archives of General Psychiatry, 12*, 63–70.

Index

Page numbers followed by an *f* or *t* indicate figures or tables.